ESSAYS ON ISSUES
IN REHABILITATION
1957-1988

ESSAYS ON ISSUES IN REHABILITATION 1957-1988

The Collected Published and Unpublished Papers of James S. Peters Ph.D., DAPA

James S. Peters II

ISBN 1-57309-121-9 (cloth   )
ISBN 1-57309-120-0 (pbk.   )

This book is dedicated to Drs. F.G. Clark, Southern University; G.R. Wells, Hartford Seminary, School of Religious Education; P.S. Shurrager, Illinois Institute of Technology; C. Rogers, University of Chicago; and H.H. Remmers, Purdue University who advised me and supported my efforts to be a student of psychology and rehabilitation.

❦

TABLE OF CONTENTS

CHAPTER ONE

THE SHELTERED WORKSHOP— A VOCATIONAL REHABILITATION RESOURCE

James S. Peters, II, Ph.D.
Bureau of Vocational Rehabilitation Connecticut
State Department of Education

The current upsurge of interest throughout this country and abroad in workshops for the disabled and in rehabilitation in general has come from a slowly developing but far-reaching social consciousness of the employment and other rehabilitation needs of the physically and mentally handicapped. The still mushrooming effects of advances in rehabilitation during World War II and later years have contributed toward a greater community awareness of the efforts being made on behalf of disabled persons, particularly in the area of rehabilitation as part of medical care. Accompanying this has been a steady growth of appreciation of the merits of vocational rehabilitation, both for disabled civilians and veterans. There has been increasing understanding of the economic and human benefits to be reaped from vocational services to persons left with physical or mental limitations as result of illness, injury or congenital conditions.

The continual success of our democratic way of life is dependent upon how sharply focused are our minds upon the tasks that lie ahead. These tasks are within the realms of medicine, engineering, law, psychology, education, etc., all of the professions. But guidance counselors, businessmen, industrialists and educators will agree with me when I say that for every doctor we need about 50 medical or laboratory technicians

---

Talk prepared for The Sheltered Workshop, Inc., Symposium, Bridgeport, Conn., January 9, 1957.

1

ESSAYS ON ISSUES IN REHABILITATION: 1957–1988

for every engineer about 100 or more electrical, chemical, etc., technicians; for every lawyer at least five or six legal secretaries, and so the story goes. We also know that in this emerging push-button society of ours it will be the trained technician who will demand respect and recognition in tomorrow's world. The white collar worker may be having his today, but the trained technician is having his tomorrow. I make no attempt to de-emphasize the important role of the white collar worker in modern society. But, I am attempting to recast our perception about the world of work so that our horizon might be broadened."

Education is a sound and necessary investment in the future well-being of our nation and its citizens. In November 1955 a committee of the White House Conference on Education, working with the problem "What Should Our Schools Accomplish," reported the following:

1. The fundamental skills of communication—reading, writing, spelling, as well as other elements of effective oral and written expression; the arithmetical and mathematical skills, including problem-solving. While schools are doing the best job in their history in teaching these skills, continuous improvement is desirable and necessary.
2. Appreciation for our democratic heritage.
3. Civic rights and responsibilities and knowledge of American institutions.
4. Respect and appreciation for human values and for the beliefs of others.
5. Ability to think and evaluate constructively and creatively.
6. Effective work habits and self-discipline.
7. Social competency as a contributing member of his family and community.
8. Ethical behavior based on a sense of moral and spiritual values.
9. Intellectual curiosity and eagerness for lifelong learning.
10. Aesthetic appreciation and self-expression in the arts.
11. Physical and mental health.
12. Wise use of time, including constructive leisure pursuits.
13. Understanding of the physical world and man's relation to it as represented through basic knowledge of the sciences.
14. An awareness of our relationships with the world community... If your education has enabled you to conceptualize and internalize most of the things enumerated above "your horizon will be broadened."

2

In order to keep our sights raised and our aspiration within the realm of reality, we must continue to be students. We must remember that in the final analysis we are responsible for ourselves. Another way of looking at this is to see ourselves, as students, ready and willing to learn and to be taught. Nevertheless, you must know that the real student is responsible for his own education. Unless he takes that responsibility, he will not become educated. A school or a college can provide the buildings, the teachers, the books and the equipment, but these are the environment of learning, not learning itself. The student must bring to his teachers an interest in learning, a respect for what the teacher can give him, a readiness to learn and a will to become educated. Without that, the teacher does all the work and the student learns merely to accommodate himself to the system by whatever means he can devise. This calls for adjustment to one's self as well as to other people. Adjustment is essential to learning how to "broaden one's horizon."

When we speak of adjustment we are talking about a psychological phenomenon which takes place in all of us. We are constantly making adjustments to personal happenings as well as social events. Though problems of adjustment are unique for each individual there are certain characteristics of the psychological living conditions of people in our culture which have general implications for the adjustment. Take the threat of an atomic war with Russia. I am sure that if a well designed questionnaire were passed among you assessing your attitudes and feelings toward this threat there would be some communality of agreement as to existence of anxiety among us and the need of having to make some adjustment. Now the degree of adjustment is not too important but the kind, positive or negative, is. When one makes a positive or good adjustment to himself he is prone to make a positive adjustment to others and to the world in which he lives.

Dr. Richard Cabot, renowned professor of medicine at Harvard during the early part of this century, names four things men lived by' work, play, love and worship. Physical defect may impair one's ability to enter into one or all of these, but there is no physical disability that can destroy our ability to do any one of them. There is no one so physically disabled that he cannot do some kind of work, play in some fashion, invest love in someone, and find some ways to worship. As long as we are human, we can enjoy these activities, no matter what limitations have been placed on us physically. This aspect of "broadening our horizon" is essential to sharing the good life here on earth.

All of us have limitations imposed upon us from without or from within. We are constantly being reminded of such as we struggle to cope with the problems of everyday living. But if I were to charge you this afternoon I would say, "Do not let these social, physical or mental limitations serve as an albatross around your neck." The world is too big and the future too bright to say that there is no niche for me in the scheme of things. I recall too vividly, during World War II while I was a student at the Hartford Seminary, an occasion when I was studying in the library and my philosophy professor came to me and inquired if I knew of any reference books on the life of George Washington Carver, the noted scientist. After I told him of several, he said "Mr. Peters, would you like to know why I want to read about Dr. Carver?" I said that I would. "Well," the professor said, "I am going to speak at a high school commencement exercise at a high school in Kansas where I taught many years ago. I am going to tell those young people who are graduating during these dreadful and uncertain times, if a malnourished, sickly slave boy who was traded for a broken down horse can 'broaden his horizon' and become one of the best known scientists of our time, there is little need for you to have fear of the future."

The world is in need of men and women who have known the pangs of deprivation and limitation. So often these entities become wings upon which we soar to greater and greater heights. We need only cite a few men of genius like socially handicapped Jesus of Nazareth, the blind poet Milton, the club-looted Lord Byron, the partially-sighted naval hero Lord Nelson, the hard-of-hearing Thomas Edison, to illustrate how greatness so often comes from suffering. I am reminded of a story that my father used to tell about the great abolitionist female, Sojourner Truth. It was at an abolitionist meeting during the dark days of the civil war when it looked as if the tide of battle were on the side of the rebel south. The meeting was being addressed by Frederick Douglass, the famous leader and orator. On this occasion Douglass's voice was lacking in vigor and fire which ordinarily stirred his audiences. Toward the end of his speech he was heard to say, "It appears that the cause of abolition of slavery is lost." A hush settled on the meeting place and for a few minutes you could hear a pin drop. Suddenly from the back of the room came a voice as pure and as clear as a bell. It said, "Douglass, is God dead?" This was the voice of Sojourner Truth, asking the question that we should ask ourselves in times of stress and strain. And the answer will be now, as it was then and will always be even unto the end of the world; no, God is not dead, but he may lie dormant within any of us unless we "broaden our horizon" and get a new vision of light, this being our cultural heritage.

❦

THE COMMUNITY'S RESPONSIBILITY TO THE DISABLED

James S. Peters, II, Ph.D.
Director, Bureau of Vocational Rehabilitation
Connecticut State Department of Education

Madam Chairman, President Lane, Officers, Members and Friends of the Tuberculosis and Health Association of the Stamford area, I am exceedingly happy to be with you this noon in order to share the beginning of a unique experience in "human relations," This great responsibility which you are undertaking, as a group, places you among that select group of mortals, to paraphrase Jesus Christ of Nazareth, who have become their "brothers' keeper." I am certain that history will be kind to all of you when such deeds are recorded in the annals of human progress as guidelines for posterity in the area of human relations. Your program will succeed for it rests upon a firm foundation of over a half century of work in tuberculosis control. Congruent with the recent announcement of the proposed retirement of the executive director of your state's program, Mable Baird, who has given 40 years of her life to this needy cause, your program has entered into a new era; an era of coordinated medical, legal, psychological, social, and economic effort to rehabilitate the disabled. It is on this phase that I wish to focus this noon.

In the year 1929, when the Connecticut State Legislature accepted the Federal Vocational Act a new opportunity of community responsibility was offered the citizens of Connecticut. This act served as a mandate by the people through their elected representatives, for professional rehabilitation personnel to prepare, where feasible, disabled individuals for return to economically gainful employment. From the year 1930 to 1934, this

---

A talk delivered at the first annual meeting of the Tuberculosis and Health Association of the Stamford area, Hugo's Restaurant, Stamford, Connecticut, Tuesday, April 30, 1957.

program functioned as a one-man operation, with Edward P. Chester, my predecessor, serving as both supervisor and counselor. From the beginning, the vocational rehabilitation operation was closely geared to the work of other private and public community welfare agencies. During those formative years, the record shows that such private organizations as your own State Tuberculosis Association cooperated in the referral of cases and the support of training programs initiated by Vocational Rehabilitation through case services. This cooperative community, interagency, effort is of a 25-year duration.

In further study of the history and perhaps, "fossil remains," of vocational rehabilitation in this great state of Connecticut there is recorded the following:

In 1935, some funds from the sale of Christmas Seals were pooled with Federal funds to finance a program of rehabilitation of the tuberculous. This program became a country "first" in the advancement of rehabilitation of the tuberculous. Mr. John W. Hekeley has received wide recognition for his pioneering work in this field.

In further recognition of the monumental work which our organization has done in the area of rehabilitation of the tuberculous, two years ago we were awarded nearly a quarter of a million dollars through the Office of Vocational Rehabilitation, Department of Health, Education and Welfare, Washington, D.C. under P.L. 565 to put into action a demonstration project of Vocational Rehabilitation for in-patient tuberculous and neuro-psychiatric cases. This program is for a three-year period and is serving as a model for the nation. Several, well-trained, rehabilitation counselors were hired to handle this work. They serve on a roving basis, all of the public institutions, and some private ones, where there are tuberculous and neuro-psychiatric patients. In a tentative attempt at evaluation of this program after a year and a half of its existence we found it necessary to put more teeth into it by upgrading John Hekeley from Supervisor of T.B. Services to Chief of Institutional Services in order that the overall program could gain from his years of rehabilitation experience with the tuberculosis program. To quote Dr. E.C. Edson, Treasurer of your association, Superintendent and Medical Director at Cedarcrest Sanitorium, "John Hekeley's service to the tuberculosis program of the State of Connecticut will be long remembered and cherished."

It is not my intention to bore you with statistics or to "brain-wash" you with the acts, overt or covert, of our Bureau but I would, however, like your indulgence while acquainting you with some significant figures that our statistical control unit shoved into my hands prior to my leaving Hartford to give this talk. After approximately twenty-five years of existence, our bureau has rehabilitated 14,000 clients. The annual number of disabled served has increased from 159 in the year 1930, to 3,409 in 1955. The number of tuberculous persons rehabilitated has increased substantially since 1938 when the special services for the tuberculous were initiated. The percentage of T.B. cases also increased; for example, in the last 5 years we have aided, through these services the return to the vocational, social and economic way of life, 1288 persons physically restricted by tuberculosis. They were trained and suitably employed. The percentage of T.B. cases rehabilitated represents approximately 26.4% of all types of disabilities.

The average cost for hospitalization in the Sanatorium today is approximately $84.00 per week. Every tuberculous person returned to employment represents a saving to society as well as to the person, as well as reasonable assurance of enabling him to maintain his restored health.

The types of professions, skills and semi-skills represented in the foregoing group of rehabilitants is greatly diversified. To mention a few— teachers, technicians (laboratory, x-ray and industrial, draftsmen), secretarial, electronics, rehabilitation counselors, medical technicians, machinists, home managers, commercial artists, toolmaker, sales, commercial workers and many others. The follow-up of these cases after closure has been gratifying.

The employer in a great many instances has expressed his approval of the quantity and quality of the rehabilitants' production and loyalty of his employee.

Now it is needless for me to say to such a well informed group as you that all this could have been accomplished by our Bureau alone. Rehabilitation is a "teamwork" affair; and the very core of teamwork has developed out of community organization; community organizations such as your own newly formed Association, organized around a common interest. Your lay and professional leadership constitute a team of workers and it is through this team working with other existing teams that the ultimate goal of rehabilitation and disease control is achieved. In order to do the functional job in rehabilitation we must be willing to lay aside old prejudices and fears in order that we might utilize every available resource in the community. There is plenty of work to be done as you well know.

As most of us have surmised, the so-called miracle drugs are greatly aiding us in the fight to control and cure tuberculosis. In a large number of tuberculosis situations chemotherapy had made an astonishing inroad into our former long-term care program, making it unnecessary, in a number of instances, for us to gear our program to traditional methods. But I say to you this noon that these newer and successful treatments should not allow us to relax our vigilance in the fight against this dreaded enemy. Chemo-therapeutic treatment has not been with us long enough for us to say the battle is well in hand; all is over but the mopping up operations; this, we can leave to the infantry—the technicians and professional people. I want to go on record as saying that the community need for tuberculosis control today is as great as it ever was. It is the responsibility of every citizen to get behind these association drives with money and labor in order that they will taste the fruit of success if we are to continue to push back the curtain of ignorance where tuberculosis is concerned. In all of your 14 area tuberculosis associations with its 42 tuberculosis committees there is a need for going beyond the all-time high of $464,600, nearly a half million dollars, raised in your 1956 campaign.

In order to bring this thinking a bit closer to you I wish to remark that according to your recent case-finding results as reported in your bulletin for April, 1957 your case-finding technique may be changed. This will include, among other things, concentration for x-ray examination among people above 45 years of age, especially those who are transients or unattached such as the skid-row addicts. Aside from this, emphasis may be given to reaching those people living in substandard crowded areas of our large cities. This is further indication of the progressive way in which your professional staff handles its job. These people are not afraid of change when such change is based on research findings.

These and other things that you are doing for the disabled transcend mere professional and lay busy work. You are demonstrating the principle of humanitarianism which is the essence of civilization. As Aristotle said so many years ago:

Man is by nature a social animal, and an individual who is unsocial naturally and not accidentally is either beneath our notice or more than human. Society is something in nature that precedes the individual. Anyone who either cannot lead the common life or is so self-sufficient as not to need to, and therefore does not partake of society, is either a beast or he is God.

꽃

SHOULD WE 'INDENTURE' REHABILITATION COUNSELORS?

James S. Peters, II, Ph.D.
Bureau of Vocational Rehabilitation Connecticut State Department of Education

I have been asked to discuss whether it is professionally desirable, ethical and feasible to require on the part of counselors who accept traineeships or trainee positions, a commitment of a given number of years of service in a particular agency or setting in return for said traineeship or training opportunity. This is a problem with which many public and private agencies are presently confronted and which others will be dealing with in the future.

Indentured servitude has been a part of the American labor scene for well over three centuries and in spite of its evil connotations has infiltrated certain aspects of those nobler professions of teaching, medicine, social work and psychology. Thus, it follows that in proposing to indenture rehabilitation counselors we are simply following the *Zeitgeist.*

James Truslow Adams in his monumental work, *The Epic of America,* writes of the motley assortment of persons that settled in the colonies during the 17th century. Among the colonists of Jamestown and Plymouth were many indentured servants and debt ridden gentlemen from England. This type of slavery differed only in degree from the more widespread institution of chattel slavery which followed. Though indentured servitude was less harsh than chattel slavery, we all know that it was just as degrading to human character, and it soon passed from the American scene as a respectable institution. However, the idea, if not the fact, has remained. In the field of medicine, for example, we witnessed fifty years ago the

Presented at Symposium on Problems and Issues in Rehabilitation Counseling, American Psychological Association Convention, Statler Hotel, New York City., September 3, 1957.

emergence of an apprentice on-the-job training type of profession which demanded that the trainee work for the master over a given period of time. Today, however, no recognized university or postgraduate training program makes such demands on the graduate. In fact, each year thousands of dollars are committed to postgraduate training of medical students with very few strings attached other than that they work in the field of medicine. There are numerous private and public grants for promising medical specialists and only in certain situations are recipients of such grants expected to work in a given institution, for a particular individual, or in a restricted area of the country. Even in residency programs, as seen in the Veterans Administration, the young medic after serving his residency becomes a free agent, that is unless he has identified too intensely with the chief of clinical services or has been overly indoctrinated in nuptial preconceptions by the head nurse.

Today, in another area, that of teacher education, we are seeing a boom in graduate scholarship offerings to promising teachers, in order to help relieve the nationwide shortage of instructors with advanced degrees. With the need for elementary and secondary teachers soaring to astronomical heights each year, most leaders in the field of education are concentrating now upon attracting and keeping bright young men and young women in public school teaching, rather than being concerned about whether they are going to work in a specific school system for a specific number of years after accepting tuition assistance. However, I must rush to point out that indenturing teachers certainly is a known practice in some local situations.

The Vocational Rehabilitation Amendments of 1954, commonly referred to as Public Law 565 of the 83rd Congress, were designed to increase to 200,000 the number of disabled persons rehabilitated each year. In order to accomplish such a task, money was appropriated through the Office of Vocational Rehabilitation to universities with approved training programs in rehabilitation counseling and scholarships up to $1,600 per year are given to interested college graduates who can qualify for the training.

In view of this present and continuing need for more and better trained personnel in rehabilitation, OVR and the several universities responsible for training, have concentrated on professional training and placement. They have not deemed it necessary to obligate scholarship recipients to working with one particular public or private agency for a given period of time.

Many deserving young men and women have heeded the call to become associated with this new program. Results of training, to date, have been excellent. The young people have shown much enthusiasm, as well as considerable insight and understanding of the work in this area in both private and public agencies. Their contribution, while too early to assess adequately at this time, is certainly bound to be of lasting benefit to the overall rehabilitation movement.

This is desirable, I believe. This is what we want. Rehabilitation counseling as a profession within the field of psychology should be encouraged to grow and to flourish as have clinical and counseling psychology in recent years.

The basic fact is that vocational rehabilitation, through public agencies, is a joint Federal and State governmental undertaking, supported by tax dollars from all citizens. Vocational rehabilitation is a community responsibility, and the community, in turn, profits from its undertakings. All, therefore, are entitled to services of individuals who have been supported financially for graduate study through training grants from the Office of Vocational Rehabilitation. Private as well as public health, education and welfare agencies should be able to profit from the training received by counselors.

But, you may say, a large number of individuals are working as rehabilitation counselors in public agencies without the advantage of the kind of graduate training which enables one to meet and accept changes that come about from new discoveries and principles. Should counselors be encouraged to seek additional training, with the aid of grants made possible under Public Law 565 and funds from the states, and then allowed to move on to another agency?

In presenting my viewpoint here, I am cognizant of the need of agencies and various communities for trained personnel in vocational rehabilitation. I am fully aware of ongoing programs which support additional training for personnel and which demand, in return for the training received, that the recipient repay the agency in service or in kind. However, I am most concerned with the individual counselor. It is my firm belief that when we indenture people we stifle growth based on individual needs and aspirations. We deny the person his basic rights as a citizen in a free society. I feel that counselors who are given opportunities for training should be not required to return to or repay their agencies. The training program for rehabilitation counseling is labyrinthine enough without saddling onto it the dictum of professional placement and/or tenure difficulties. We hardly need to arouse additional anxieties to add to those already created by the numerous expectancies of the role which the rehabilitation counselor plays. In my opinion, therefore, the philosophy of indenture is archaic and can best be symbolized as a "cultural lag" or a pre-professional albatross.

In the area of human engineering we are particularly interest in freeing the individual of restrictive obligations so that he might become self-actualizing, with a minimum of impediments to growth and development in a free society. It is possible that by not indenturing rehabilitation counselors we are respecting human worth and dignity, two basic aspects of healthy personality functioning.

This is all well and good, but the administrator may still be faced with the immediate and practical problem of acquiring better trained personnel, with providing additional training or educational opportunities for employees who do not meet desired standards for professional vocational rehabilitation counselors.

If the complete freeing of the individual from the obligation to return to or to repay the agency is impractical, then, perhaps each agency should be encouraged to evaluate its individual situation in the light of what the counselor is contributing or has contributed to its program. In this way training assistance is based on meritorious service of personnel rather than solely on the needs of the agency for better trained personnel.

A good worker deserves a reward with no strings attached.

❦

CHAPTER FOUR

REHABILITATION COUNSELOR PREPARATION AND PROFESSIONAL GROWTH OPPORTUNITIES

James S. Peters, II, Ph.D.
Bureau of Vocational Rehabilitation
Connecticut State Department of Education

A review of the development of our rehabilitation movement reveals a steady expansion of social services, and particularly rehabilitation services, based upon the total needs of disabled individuals and groups in our various communities. As professional advances have been made and utilized in the area of rehabilitation, the role of the rehabilitation counselor has changed. At the present time, counselor preparation is in a fluid state.

Systematic rehabilitation services for handicapped individuals are of relatively recent origin. The first nationwide public effort in rehabilitation was the vocational rehabilitation training program initiated in 1918 for disabled veterans of World War I. In part as a result of early experiences in that program and the general interest stimulated in restoring disabled individuals to gainful employment, the first legislation providing for state-federal vocational rehabilitation for disabled civilians was passed in 1920. Up to the outbreak of World War II there was a gradual expansion of the state-federal program for physically and mentally disabled individuals. This same period also witnessed the development of multi-service rehabilitation programs based upon the complete needs of the disabled in the integration of specialized professional efforts into coordinated rehabilitation centers.

An address given at the Office of Vocational Rehabilitation, Region I, Orientation Training Institute, Boston University Conference Center, Osgood Hill, North Andover, Massachusetts, Friday, November 22, 1957.

World War II gave impetus to three dominant influences which exerted a marked effect upon the field of rehabilitation and facilitated a rapid expansion of existing programs and the establishment of new and more varied facilities and services. The first of these was the reconditioning and rehabilitation activities set up during the course of the war by the various armed forces. These activities demonstrated that by employing appropriate rehabilitation measures and techniques many disabled servicemen could be returned to active duty, while others who were unable to return to duty could be released to their specific communities in an improved physical and mental condition which accelerated their adjustment to an active and useful civilian life.

The second influence was the dramatic demonstration to employers as well as to many disabled individuals, that through selective placement handicapped workers could take their places in industry and make significant contributions to national defense. This served the purpose of opening the doors of industry to handicapped workers and brought to national attention the vast reservoir of unused but potentially useful manpower represented by the thousands of handicapped individuals in the population.

The third influence was the program of vocational rehabilitation of disabled veterans of World War II provided by Public Law 16, passed in 1943, and the expanded and improved programs for civilians provided in the same year by Public Law 113. The momentum given the rehabilitation movement by the accelerated program sponsored by the Veterans Administration and other governmental and voluntary agencies resulted in the marked growth of rehabilitation facilities. This growing demand to enlarge the scope of rehabilitation was reflected in the passage in 1954 of Public Law 565 by Congress to provide greatly increased facilities and personnel to meet the total rehabilitation needs of disabled individuals in everyday life.

Increasing public acceptance of health and welfare services has brought changes in the purpose for which such services are rendered. The concepts of counselor functioning, and hence counselor preparation, have gradually responded to the change in public attitude toward rehabilitation of the disabled.

The rapid expansion of both public and voluntary rehabilitation programs has serious implications for many aspects of current rehabilitation efforts, the most obvious one being the need for more trained personnel. Among the urgently needed workers is the rehabilitation counselor. Expanding programs, of necessity, have developed new services and operations which had not been considered heretofore. Accord-

14

ingly, the very scope and nature of rehabilitation counselor activities have expanded concurrently with the development of the programs.

Rehabilitation includes a series of services which aim to conserve, develop, or restore the ability of disabled persons so that they may become economically independent by having an opportunity to achieve a satisfactory level of employability. Regardless of the setting in which the rehabilitation counselor may work or the professional title by which he may be known, his essential role is to see that these services are provided directly or otherwise, in an orderly and effective manner. The role, the functions, and the responsibilities of the rehabilitation counselor demand knowledge and skills and personal characteristics especially keyed to serve the disabled clientele. This is the client-centered approach, but not non-directive.

In attempting to outline the areas of content to the professional education of the rehabilitation counselor, several things become evident. First, it is a fact that such preparation must draw heavily upon a number of well-established disciplines, knowledge, and skills. Second, it is necessary that the rehabilitation counselor learn the nature, philosophy, and practice of other professional disciplines with which he will be working, so that he may make appropriate use of these services in related fields and participate as an effective member of various clinical, consulting and community rehabilitation teams.

Legislative Aspects of Rehabilitation

A great deal of the progress being made in the rehabilitation of the handicapped is the direct or indirect result of state and federal legislation. Some of this legislation has had the expansion of rehabilitation as its announced objective, but rehabilitation efforts have also been greatly influenced by general health and welfare legislation. In almost any setting in which the rehabilitation counselor works, his day-to-day activities and the general direction of his efforts are affected by legislation. Therefore, the professional education of the rehabilitation counselor should include a study of important pertinent legislation.

Human Development and Behavior

The scope of counselor education in the area of human development and behavior will depend largely upon the extent to which the needs of the trainee have been met by prior training and experience. Areas such as growth, maturation, learning, emotional development, motivation, individual differences and personality adjustment are essential areas of exploration in rehabilitation counselor training and in all of the disciplines which are related to counselor education.

15

Medical Aspects of Rehabilitation

The physical and mental needs of the patient influence the entire rehabilitation process and should be clearly understood before a vocational rehabilitation plan is instituted. Rehabilitation counselor education includes a comprehensive survey of the functions and services of medicine in rehabilitation. The counselor should be familiar with elementary medical terminology in order to have the tools with which to interpret medical reports. Familiarity with some of the basic diagnostic, evaluative and therapeutic procedures is desirable. He should have an appreciation of the value of medical and psychiatric information pertaining to a client. The counselor should also be aware of the implications of disabilities for vocational and occupational adjustment.

Cultural and Psychological Aspects of Disability

The curriculum of rehabilitation counselor education should survey the impact of cultural and psycho-social influences upon the disabled. These influences are a part of each person's environment. Impacts—such as the disabled person's family, his educational status, special influences of ethnic and religious groups, variations in customs and stresses of urban or rural living, effects of disablement in early life and of results of institutional living, all are elements in the environment of the disabled which should be surveyed.

Psychological Evaluation

Almost every aspect of the work of the rehabilitation counselor has significant psychological implications. Therefore, rehabilitation counseling requires psychological understanding, knowledge and skill. Basic to these are an understanding of human behavior and adjustment, and of the techniques for gaining and assimilating this understanding.

Counseling Techniques

The rehabilitation counselor may assume different roles in the rehabilitation process. Inherent in all these roles is the counselor's responsibility to interpret the rehabilitation process to the client, discuss with him the various stages of rehabilitation and secure pertinent information in a face-to-face relationship.

Occupational and Educational Information

The collection, development and uses of occupational, educational and related information by the rehabilitation counselor is done in a different orientation from that of the general counselor. While much of general counseling preparation offers useful direction in rehabilitation counseling education, the latter deals with a specialized approach related to specific needs of the client. The limitations of a given client require a different emphasis in selecting the job or school to fit his residual capacities and needs. The very nature of the client's disability requires a more precise focusing of training.

Community Resources

In order to meet the varied needs of the client, the rehabilitation counselor must know his community's resources and be able to make discriminating use of them. Community resources include agencies and individuals. Examples are employment offices, diagnostic and treatment clinics, churches, service clubs and community-spirited individuals. The potentialities of any resource to meet a rehabilitation need are frequently beyond its stated purpose. This is particularly true in rural areas, characterized by the absence of well-organized voluntary agencies.

Placement and Follow-Up

Rehabilitation counselors need instruction on how to assist the disabled person in obtaining suitable employment. Employment may be secured by personal efforts of the client with the assistance of the rehabilitation counselor or placement agencies in the community such as the State Employment Service.

Research and Statistics

The rehabilitation counselor should bear in mind that he should be familiar with the statistical and research methods for counselors to the fullest extent that his training and job requirements will allow. With several courses in statistics and research available in most training programs, the typical rehabilitation counselor should have completed at least elementary statistics and a course in methods of research.

Supervised Experience

In addition to his academic training, the education of a rehabilitation counselor should include participation in a systematic program of supervised practice. Such practice is in many respects the most important phase of the rehabilitation counseling training. Without it the trainee could be partially or totally incapable of assuming an effective role as a counselor, regardless of the amount of academic preparation he had completed.

❦

Rehabilitation Today

James S. Peters, II, Ph.D.
Director, Bureau of Vocational Rehabilitation
Connecticut State Department of Education

It is a pleasure, as well as a privilege, to be with you this afternoon and to bring greetings from the Connecticut State Department of Education and the Bureau of Vocational Rehabilitation. The members of the State Board of Education, Governor, members of the State Legislature and Congressmen are all interested in the pervasive problems of rehabilitation. This interest has been amply demonstrated by the monetary contribution which the State and the Federal Governments have made to our Bureau for the biennium. The combined appropriation comes to well over a million dollars. This, coupled with grant-in-aid money coming from the Office of Vocational Rehabilitation on a matching basis for approved projects in rehabilitation conducted in the State, means that close to two-million dollars will be spent on rehabilitation in the State of Connecticut through our agency during the next two years.

Now it is not my intention to laud the program of the Bureau of Vocational Rehabilitation this afternoon for the 967 rehabilitants for fiscal 1956-57 speak for themselves; but rather, I am here to congratulate you for your interest in a most deserving group of our citizenry, the handicapped.

The accomplishments of vocational rehabilitation in Connecticut are attested to by His Excellency Governor Abraham Ribicoff in his message to our Bureau in commemoration of our Silver Anniversary last year. His message is as follows:

> The achievements of Vocational Rehabilitation during
> the past 25 years have made it commonplace for the

A talk delivered before Hartford Chapter of Civitan, Friday, November 29, 1957, Hotel Bond.

disabled person to work successfully beside the able-bodied individual in Connecticut factories, stores and other establishments.

Wise employers find that it is not only a good deed but good business to hire the disabled. The Bureau of Vocational Rehabilitation of the State Department of Education is proud of its quarter-century record of assisting more than 14,000 disabled person to become self-supporting.

Behind this accomplishment stands the cooperation of many employers and community agencies, and above all the courage of the disabled persons themselves.

Rehabilitation of the disabled taps a new reservoir of manpower. It turns persons who have been assisted from tax revenues into active producers of goods, services and greater tax revenues. It provides the dignity of self-support to men and women who are anxious to earn weekly pay checks.

Most important, it gives these people a sense of creating and a joy in living.

Upon this occasion, I am happy to congratulate the public and private agencies, the business establishments and the labor organizations which play a part in Vocational Rehabilitation work in Connecticut.

Rehabilitation

Rehabilitation is the restoration of the handicapped to the maximum physical, mental, social, vocational and economic usefulness of which they are capable.

To Whom is Vocational Rehabilitation Available?

Any handicapped person sixteen years of age or older, residing in Connecticut, who can be reasonably expected to profit by rehabilitation services should apply for consideration.

Persons with disabilities resulting from birth, disease, accident or from emotional causes are served. These include arm and leg deformities, amputations, heart ailments, tuberculosis, hearing, speech and eye defects, and many other handicapping conditions.

The Vocational Rehabilitation Process

The process of vocational rehabilitation is designed to provide services to develop, preserve, or restore the ability of the disabled to perform remunerative work. Each disabled person served receives the combination of services which meets his or her individual need. These services may include diagnostic examinations, counseling, medical services, prostheses, training, maintenance, transportation, tools, job finding, and follow-up.

Historical Background

In 1929, the Connecticut State Legislature accepted the Federal Vocational Rehabilitation Act and made a small appropriation for the inauguration of a state program of vocational rehabilitation. From 1930 to 1934, the program functioned as a one-man operation, with Mr. Edward P. Chester acting both as supervisor and counselor. In 1934, some temporary emergency funds from the government enabled Mr. Chester to employ five counselors. But, by the end of 1935, these funds were no longer available and the program returned to its one-man operation.

In 1935, some funds from the sale of Christmas Seals were pooled with federal funds to finance a program of rehabilitation of the tuberculous. This program became a country "first" in the advancement of rehabilitation of the tuberculous. Mr. John W. Hekeley has received wide recognition for his pioneering work in this field. By 1940, upon the Bureau's tenth anniversary, another counselor was added, making a total statewide staff of three workers. In 1941, the Bureau with its small staff initiated another country "first." This was its pioneering work in the "team approach," which led to the inauguration of the Rehabilitation Clinic, then widely known as the "Man-Salvage Clinic."

Gradually funds were increased, primarily as a result of enactment of Federal amendments in 1943. At that time offices were opened in New Haven and Bridgeport. In 1944 offices were added at Hartford, Norwich and Waterbury.

After twenty-five years and the achievement of 14,000 completed rehabilitations, the Bureau has two district and eight local offices scattered in the key communities of the State. These offices are located in Hartford, Bridgeport, New Haven, Stamford, Waterbury, Danbury, Newton, Meriden, Norwich, and New Britain. The annual number of handicapped served has increased form 159 in the year 1930, to 3,409 in 1955.

Vocational Rehabilitation Services

1. *Diagnostic Services*: To determine extent of disability and work capacity through medical, psychiatric, and psychological examinations.
2. *Counseling*: To help the disabled person select and attain the right job objective, through careful study of all factors involved.
3. *Medical Services*: To help bring back or improve the person's ability to work.
4. *Prostheses; Medical Appliances*: To fulfill need for physical aids such as artificial limbs, braces, and hearing aids.
5. *Training*: To develop skills to do the right job.
6. *Maintenance; Transportation*: To provide means for board, room, and travel during training, if necessary.
7. *Tools, Equipment, Licenses*: To meet needs of certain jobs, when ready for work.
8. *Job Finding*: To help find the right job, when ready for work.
9. *Follow-Up*: To make sure the rehabilitated worker has adjusted to his job, both to his own satisfaction and that of his employer.

Now that we have reviewed some of the organizational and program features of vocational rehabilitation in Connecticut, let me say a few words about our field personnel—the rehabilitation counselors.

The rehabilitation counselor is a person trained in the technique of vocational rehabilitation and all that this entails. He is, or is becoming, an expert in the following areas:

1. Legislative aspects of rehabilitation
2. Human development and behavior
3. Medical aspects of rehabilitation
4. Cultural and psycho-social aspects of disability
5. Psychological evaluation
6. Counseling techniques
7. Occupational and educational information
8. Community resources
9. Placement and follow-up
10. Research and statistics
11. Supervised experience

In outlining the areas of competency of the rehabilitation counselor several things become evident. First is the fact that the rehabilitation counselor must draw heavily upon a number of established disciplines for certain knowledge and skills. Second, it is important that the rehabilitation counselor acquire additional knowledge and skills peculiar to the needs of the disabled. Third, it is important that the rehabilitation counselor learn the nature, philosophy, and practice of other professional disciplines with which he will be working, so that he can make appropriate use of services in these related fields and participate as an effective member of various clinical, consulting, or community rehabilitation teams.

The team concept is of paramount importance in vocational rehabilitation. Dr. Lloyd H. Lofquist in his recent book entitled *Vocational Counseling with the Physically Handicapped* has this to say:

> To best utilize all resources, there has been increasing emphasis on the team concept and the total rehabilitation idea in hospital methodology. There is growing recognition of the fact that large expenditures of professional time and money in treatment are of little ultimate value unless the patient has found it possible to implement a vocational plan that is consonant with his physical and mental condition and permits him to follow medical recommendations. As a consequence, the vocational counseling psychologist has been given a critical position in the total treatment plan.

It is interesting to note that "Teamwork in serving the Handicapped" is the theme of the September 1957 issue of the Employment Security Review which is published by the U.S. Department of Labor, Bureau of Employment Security, U.S. Employment Service. In a most interesting article by Cyrus G. Flanders of the Connecticut State Employment Service, entitled, "Cooperation—The Persistent Kind," is the following about a rehabilitation case:

> In spite of these severe handicaps, John has become a well-adjusted individual and is making good in a job where he has established an excellent attendance record. This all came about because of cooperation—close cooperation—between the Bureau of Vocational Rehabilitation and the Employment Service over a long discouraging period.

Cooperation is the essential ingredient in the "team concept" to which rehabilitation agencies are committed.

Let us now consider some of the facts about disabled people in this country and what can be done for them through rehabilitation.

I. How Many People in the United States Require Vocational Rehabilitation?

1. Projecting preliminary results or an extensive, long-term study in City, begun in 1954 and to be completed in 1959, against the national population, it appears that there are *approximately 2,230,000 physically handicapped adults who are feasible of rehabilitation* to the point of remunerative employment.

2. However, nearly half of this group will find employment after rehabilitation only in sheltered workshops.

3. *Each year an additional 250,000* disabled persons *come to need vocational rehabilitation.*

II. What are the Main Causes of Disability Among Americans?

1. *Chronic disease* (which includes such diseases as heart disease, tuberculosis, mental illness, multiple sclerosis, Parkinson's Disease, epilepsy, diabetes, cancer, cerebral palsy, arthritis and various eye disorders) accounts for 88% of all disabling conditions.

Occupational accidents account for 5%; *home, highway and all other accidents* account for 5%, and *congenital conditions* account for the remaining 2%.

III. Is Physical Disability Only a Problem of Old Age?

No.

1. *Disability is no respector of age.*

2. *Rheumatic fever, cerebral palsy, epilepsy, poliomyelitis,* for the most part, *cripple the very young.*

3. *Tuberculosis attacks heavily during the productive years of life.*

4. The chronic diseases, such as those listed in Question II, take their toll in middle or later life.

5. *Nevertheless, the greatest amount of disability is found among older persons*; in a 1949 survey of disability, 39% of the 2,000,000 persons aged 14-64 whose disabilities had lasted 7 months or longer were 55-64 years of age. When the study was repeated in 1950, the percentage was almost the same—42%.

6. On any given day, 1 in every 7 men and women aged 65 or more is disabled, and 4 out of 7 of those (8% of all aged

persons) are disabled because of major chronic diseases or impairments. Their disability rate is about 2 1/2 times as large as that for the total population.

IV. What are the Public Costs of Disability?

1. *To provide maintenance and medical care for disabled people* through public assistance programs is now *costing the public about $537,000,000 annually.*

    a. In three programs authorized by the Congress, estimated annual payments to recipients are totaling:

        (1) About $73,000,000 annually for Aid to the Blind;

        (2) About $165,000,000 annually for Aid to the Permanently and Totally Disabled;

        (3) About $128,000,000 annually for Aid to Dependent Children in families where one or both of the parents is disabled and unable to support their children.

    b. Payments to disabled persons through General Assistance programs are estimated to be about $171,000,000 each year.

V. Does Rehabilitation Pay?

Yes!

1. *By reducing cost of Public Assistance.* Some of the disabled people aided by Public Assistance programs *can* be rehabilitated. Through the State-Federal Vocational Rehabilitation program, a public service to prepare physically or mentally disabled persons for employment and place them in suitable jobs, administered by the Office of Vocational Rehabilitation of the Department of Health, Education, and Welfare, 57,981 persons were rehabilitated in 1955. Of the 57,981 persons rehabilitated during 1955, *11,600 (1 out of 5) were receiving some public assistance.*

    a. These 11,600 persons *had been costing the taxpayers* at the estimated rate of *$9.6 million per year* in assistance payments.

    b. With their rehabilitation completed, they are now productive members of the community and *will earn an estimated $21,000,000 in the first year after rehabilitation* (based on the average earnings of all rehabilitants in 1955).

    c. The estimated $7.7 million spent to rehabilitate these

people is only about 80% of what it would cost to maintain them at public expense for a year; however, they will continue their earnings, as a consequence of their rehabilitation, for many years.

2. *What is the Manpower Gain to the Nation?*

a. The *57,981 persons rehabilitated in 1955 contributed about 11,000,000 man days annually to our Nation's productivity.*

3. *What is the Economic Gain to the Nation?*

a. The first-year *earnings of the 57,981 persons rehabilitated during 1955* through the State-Federal Vocational Rehabilitation Program alone *contributed $105,000,000 to the economic wealth of the Nation.*

4. *What is the Return from the Government Investment?*

a. In 1955 the total program cost of the State-Federal program of vocational rehabilitation services under Section 2 (basic support) of the Vocational Rehabilitation Act was:

Total	$38,636,578
Federal share	23,999,944
State share	14,636,634

Program cost under Section 2 of the Vocational Rehabilitation Act includes administration, counseling and guidance, medical service, job training, occupational tools and equipment, job placement and other services to clients, and expenditures for the establishment of rehabilitation facilities and workshops.

b. In one year, the persons rehabilitated by this program will pay *$8,500,000 to the Federal Government in Federal income taxes*, plus an undetermined but large amount of State and local taxes.

c. *At this rate, within 3 years they will pay back the total Federal funds invested in the Vocational Rehabilitation Program during 1955.*

VI. How Many People Were Rehabilitated In 1956?

1. In fiscal 1956, a record number of 66,273 disabled persons alone were rehabilitated to useful employment-an increase of 14% above the 57,981 rehabilitated in 1955. The costs for Section 2 (basic support) for that year were $48 million

(Federal-$30 million; State-$18 million). These increases indicate the rate at which both the Federal and State governments are increasing their efforts.

For the second consecutive time, a new record number of disabled people were restored to useful work through the public program of vocational rehabilitation during the fiscal year that ended June 30. The 1957 record was 71,570 persons rehabilitated. This was 5,274 over the 1956 record of 66,296. Miss Mary E. Switzer, Director of the Office of Vocational Rehabilitation said the 1957 figures are based on reports from State vocational rehabilitation agencies which operate in partnership with the Federal Government, and from private agencies which have received some support through OVR.

Public agencies placed 70,939 persons in jobs after helping them to overcome their disabilities, and an additional 631 were established in employment through projects developed cooperatively with voluntary groups. An additional 145,000 were receiving rehabilitation services from State agencies as the fiscal year ended. In time, most of these persons are expected to be restored to productive employment. "Although the increase over last year's record was not as great as had been expected," Miss Switzer said, "it was encouraging since 41 of the 52 States and territories showed increases in the number rehabilitated."

It is estimated that the 70,939 men and women rehabilitated through the State-Federal program will increase their annual earnings from $18.9 million to about $137.6 million, in their first full year of employment, and add 109 million man-hours to the Nation's production potential.

Among those rehabilitated during the year were some 3,500 persons who entered the short-supply professional fields of education, medicine and engineering. About 8,700 went into skilled trades and 6,100 into agriculture. Most of the others are in managerial, sales, or service jobs, or in unskilled work. About 53,000 of those rehabilitated were unemployed at the time they began to receive services. Some 14,000 had been dependent on public assistance, receiving financial aid of $11.4 million a year. The total one-time cost of rehabilitating these persons was $11.1 million. The others were in part-time, unsafe or unsuitable work when their rehabilitation was begun.

As you can see, the voluntary health organizations also constitute an ongoing part of our growing rehabilitation movement. They illuminate the broadness of our total rehabilitation approach, projecting innumerable creative ideas and ideals into this important area of human relations. All of us are dedicated to the proposition that "the handicapped" is an individual and therefore in need of personal and social orientation as well as physical restoration. This is why so many lay and professionals are needed in the rehabilitation process.

In conclusion, I wish to reiterate that in aiding the disabled you are helping the cause of freedom and human dignity; two capstones of our democratic heritage.

❦

CHAPTER SIX

REHABILITATION—PROFESSION, SCIENCE, OR ART?

James S. Peters, II, Ph.D.
Bureau of Vocational Rehabilitation
Connecticut State Department of Education

Mr. Chairman, professors, members of Sigma Theta Psi, and visiting friends; it is with distinct pleasure and pride that I return to Springfield College this evening to give, what may be called, the third annual initiation lecture of the Society of Sigma Theta Psi, graduate rehabilitation society. My heartfelt thanks and gratitude go to both students and faculty advisors who thought that I should be invited back to this rostrum where I held forth a year ago.

I must admit that this second invitation is soothing to the ego, for I have plenty in my cosmos, but I ask you, aren't we taking this personal symbol of honor a bit too far? I recall vividly the masterful inspirational lecture that my good friend, Dr. Isadore Sheerer, gave here two years ago to mark the rounding of this society. It was a gala and glorious occasion and Ike Sheerer had all of us, students and faculty alike, hanging onto his every word. He signaled the theme of our society's ultimate objective—scientific and professional endeavor. It is my sincere hope that future initiations will find me in the audience or playing a minor role in the initiation ceremony, like serving punch.

This evening I have chosen the subject for discussing with you, Rehabilitation—Profession, Science, or Art? This poses a crucial question for educators, administrators and other persons dealing with rehabilitation personnel and I doubt seriously if any of us has the answer. We may dismiss the question by one of three ways:

Third annual initiation lecture, Society of Sigma Theta Psi, Springfield College, Springfield, Massachusetts, January 23, 1958.

1. Denying that such a question as to distinction exists.
2. Acknowledging existence of the question as to distinction but seeing it as being inconsequential.
3. By recognizing existence of the question as to distinction and at the same time making some attempt to come to grip with it.

I have chosen the third alternative; the recognition of the existence of such a question as to distinction and in the next few minutes I will make a beginning, and I wish to emphasize, only a beginning, to deal with it.

My general thesis, Rehabilitation—Profession, Science, or Art question is a myth, and a logical synthesis or fusion of the biological and social sciences with the healing arts culminates in the rehabilitation profession or professions. Take Sections 2 and 3 of Article I of your own Constitution, for example. Section 2 reads:

> The purpose of this society shall be to foster high scholarships, stimulate research and scientific interest, and integrate graduate students from all areas in the field of rehabilitation.

Section 3 reads:

> The activities of the Society shall be in keeping with its purposes, to stimulate professional growth and development, aid in public education and information, engage in activities which meet community needs in the area of rehabilitation and to aid in organization of additional chapters of the Society.

In viewing the purposes and activities of your Society we conceptualize a synthesis of both scientific and professional endeavor. If this be the trend or direction of rehabilitation, support of a kind is given our thesis.

Now in order to pinpoint this material let us consider what a profession is, and also its criteria.[1]

On the Definition of a Profession

There have been many attempts to define a profession. None, however have succeeded in satisfying everyone. Some writers disclaim the possi-

---

[1] article by Leonard C. Kercher, "Who is Eligible for Torch?" The Torch, Vol. XXX, July, 1957, No. 3, pp. 3-11.

bility, and some even the desirability of such a definition. M. L. Cogan reflects these views in the following quotations from his analysis of the problem

> To define a "profession" is to invite controversy. ... so many advantages have accrued to profession, so many claims to it are made by so many people, that the cutting edge of a definition—be it ever so blunt—is almost sure to draw cries of protest from many aspirants to the title. Frances P. DeLancy states that it is impossible to locate a satisfactory definition. She asserts that an effort to make a satisfactory inventory of the characteristics must become arbitrary... There is no absolute definition of profession.
> Some of the writers most notable for their interest in the analysis of profession simply refuse to venture a definition. Outstanding representatives of these are Alexander Carr-Saunders and P.A. Wilson who, after extensive treatment of the characteristics in a greater or lesser degree, approach more or less clearly to the condition of a profession.

Such statements as these serve to drive home the conviction that a general definition of profession satisfactory to everyone is probably impossible. It seems unlikely, moreover, that further research would alter this conclusion.

Criteria of Professional

To clarify the concept, profession or professional, we familiarized ourselves with the criteria advanced by authorities in the field for judging the merits of an occupational group's claim to professional status. Considerable agreement among writers concerning these criteria is evident. Here we shall take note of the five most emphasized criteria encountered in our study.

I. Professional activity is intellectual and responsible in character. Stressed quite generally and emphatically in the literature is the intellectual character of professional work and the large measure of personal responsibility it entails. Such statements as the following abound.

> The first mark of a profession is that the activities involved are essentially intellectual in character.

The Professional takes full responsibility for the results of his efforts and activities.

...it is the nature of a profession that it bases its technique of operation upon principles rather than upon rule-of-thumb procedure or simple routine procedures.

A true profession, it thus appears, involves responsible brain work. True professional behavior is intellectually creative. It is characterized by an intellectual approach to an understanding and mastery of problems. It calls for judgment, involves responsible individual planning and performance (rather than routine rule-of-thumb procedures), and implies an understanding of the theoretical structure underlying the vocational function.

A second criterion arises logically from this first

II. A profession is based on a body of general and specialized knowledge, and possesses "educationally communicable techniques."

There is wide authoritative consensus also on this criterion. It has long been recognized as a mark of professional status in a vocation. Abraham Flexner, writing over four decades ago, had this to say on the point in general.

Despite differences of opinion about details, the members of a given profession are pretty well agreed as to the specific objects that a profession seeks to fulfill, and the specific kinds of skill that the practitioner of the profession must master in order to obtain the object in question. On this basis men arrive at an understanding as to the amount and quality of training, general and specific, which should precede admission into a professional school, as to the content and length of the professional course. These formulations are meant to exclude from professions those incapable of pursuing them in a large, free and responsible way; and to make sure that those potentially capable are so instructed as to get fullest possible benefit from the training provided.

III. A profession has practical objectives.

An emphasis on practical objectives in professional activity is likewise evident in authoritative writing. A profession, we are told, invariably points towards the fulfillment of a specific practical purpose. It must move, it appears, from mere study and acquisition of knowledge to application and practice.

No profession can be merely academic and theoretic; the professional man must have an absolutely definite and practical objective.

> A huge preponderance of the opinions surveyed for this report tends to establish that practical application of skills is inseparable from the idea of profession. Mere study and investigation is precluded and strong emphasis is placed upon practical pursuits and the vocational application of knowledge to public uses as opposed to amateurish pursuits.

IV. The prime motive of a profession is altruistic service. Wide consensus prevails also that altruistic service is an important criterion of a profession. Not monetary gain nor personal acclaim, but devotion to the service of others is regarded as the prime measure of true professional success.

> The professional worker's chief desire is to render service. To improve man's welfare is the end to which the professional worker devotes his career.
> The essence of a profession is that though men enter it for a livelihood, the measure of their success is the service which they perform, not the gains which they amass.
> The profession serving the vital needs of man, considers its first ethical imperative to be altruistic service to the client.

Altruistic service thus appears to be a guiding principle of true professional conduct. No doubt this ideal is compromised by many in practice, and by some abandoned altogether. Commercialism deeply infects some in the most ethical of professions, and there are those who prostitute music, art, and even religion, for crass monetary ends. But surely these are the regrettable exceptions rather than the rule.

V. A profession moves toward internal organization and self-government.

Another criterion usually considered a *mark* of a profession is that of self-organization. The specialized nature of professional knowledge and practice draws practitioners in a given field together for the purpose of establishing standards of practice and also for determining the requirements in formal education, experience and test results for admission to practice. This criterion is likewise widely recognized.

Another earmark of a profession is that its members organize associations to maintain and improve its services. The associations promote a high standard of professional character and honorable practice.

True professional behavior is subordination of inclinations, appetites, and ambitions of individuals to rules of an organization, which has as its object to promote the performance of functions.

One of the criteria against which to measure the professionalism of a vocation is the degree of group consciousness and integration.

…one of the indications that an occupation is becoming a profession is a concerted movement along members to establish and to maintain group discipline, that is, to uphold the ethical values involved.

Self-organization, and self-discipline through group-sanctioned standards, appears to be a valid and useful criterion for judging the professional status of a vocational group.

❣

CHAPTER SEVEN

RECENT DEVELOPMENTS IN VOCATIONAL REHABILITATION COUNSELING

James S. Peters, II, Ph.D.
Bureau of Vocational Rehabilitation
Connecticut State Department of Education

I have been asked by my good friend and former department head, Dr. Seth Arsonian, to speak on *Recent Developments in Vocational Rehabilitation Counseling*- I am happy to see that the topic has been restricted to counseling for this is the area of rehabilitation which I am best qualified by training, experience, and yes, temperament, to speak to. Then, too, as psychological counselors we have more than a mild concern about counseling in rehabilitation, we have a vested interest.

Vocational counseling and guidance has been an integral part of the rehabilitation process since the inception of the federal program of vocational rehabilitation. The program by the Federal Government for the vocational rehabilitation of persons disabled in industry or otherwise and their return to civilian employment was inaugurated on June 2, 1920. Although this date is important in the history and development of the vocational rehabilitation program, it should not be considered as the starting point nor the beginning of the program. The history of the rehabilitation movement begins with the attitudes held by primitive people regarding the physically deformed.

Early historical accounts tell of the killing, abandoning, and ridiculing of the crippled, blind, infirm, and aged. The fact that these unfortunates were unable to contribute to the group in its struggle for survival probably gave rise to the superstitious beliefs that developed concerning them.

Paper presented at Seminar on Trends and Problems in Guidance and Counseling, Springfield College, Massachusetts, June 26, 1958.

35

Physical defectives were believed to be possessed with evil powers, and thus fear resulted in an attitude of intolerance and contempt toward all the physically substandard. This universal feeling persisted for centuries, and although the practice of doing away with all those who were disabled ceased early in the Christian Era, the intolerant attitude continued. This is illustrative of the fact, often cited, that emotion and prejudice can survive for an incredibly long time after their logical bases (if they ever existed) have been removed. Professor Alport has made this point quite clear in his monumental work on *The Nature of Prejudice.*

It was not until as late as the eighteenth century that this spirit of intolerance to the physically handicapped gave way to a constructive attitude. This change in attitudes was fostered by an English orthopedic surgeon who stated that it would be wise to educate and treat disabled people. This idea was accepted and carried out first in England, and resulted in the rounding of several institutions devoted to the care of the blind and of the crippled.

In the course of events it was natural that the people in the American colonies should have many of the same attitudes as their European forefathers. Physically impaired were first thought to be bewitched, and later were simply neglected. However, the rise of modern orthopedic surgery in the nineteenth century resulted in the establishment of special institutions in the United States for crippled children. The Newington Home and Hospital in Connecticut is one such example. The success of these early institutions brought about a realization of the need for further and more adequate facilities, and in the latter part of the nineteenth century and early part of the twentieth, the U.S. Congress made several land grants to western states for special institutions to care for deaf, dumb and blind people. In 1893 Boston established an industrial school for crippled and deformed children with vocational training as its primary objective. In 1897 Minnesota took the lead and make the first direct state provision for medical care for crippled children.

By the early part of the present century, public opinion had become definitely crystallized as to the needs of the physically disabled as a group, but it remained for private agencies to point the way to a constructive solution of the problem. Among these organizations were the New York Institute for the Crippled and Disabled; the Cleveland Association for Crippled and Disabled; and the Service League for the Handicapped in Chicago. Correspondingly, numerous social agencies had also begun to turn their attention to the special problems and needs of the disabled. Major activities and functions of these groups, in relation to the physically handicapped, centered around the securing of therapeutic treatment and finding employment, and in providing artificial appliances and special job opportunities for them.

In the evolution of the rehabilitation movement, one of the most important factors that sped up the development of a constructive rehabilitation program for the disabled was the alarming growth of the problem. The great expansion in methods of manufacturing by machinery and the speeding up of transportation, with consequent disabling accidents, brought about a condition which demanded attention. Samuel Gompers and the American Federation of Labor were active in focusing attention on these conditions. Concern for the worker disabled in industry resulted in the passage, beginning in 1911, or a series of acts by the states for the purpose of compensating the disabled for injuries received while at work. In a comparatively short period of time it was generally conceded all over the country that the worker was entitled to compensation for injuries received while at work. Experience in the administration of workman's compensation laws soon demonstrated that money benefits to injured workers were not sufficient in all cases to ameliorate their condition nor to lessen the effects of physical disability. Compensation benefits were in themselves inadequate since they did not provide a margin whereby the disabled worker could fit himself for employment when his physical disability prevented his return to work.

Also, it was discovered that few disabled persons, having been barred from their customary lines of employment, were able on their own initiative to adjust themselves to new vocations.

Furthermore, facilities in the United States for retraining were for the most part not of such a nature as to enable the adult himself to secure the kind of training he need most. It became clear that the injured worker is entitled to something more than money compensation for his injury and that the interest of the community is advanced by giving him further assistance. It was deemed to be in the public interest that the injured worker be rendered fit again to engage in remunerative employment. It was also agreed that the service is clearly an obligation and responsibility of the state—a public function, rather than a matter of private interest or philanthropy. It was seen that a complete and adequate social program for the disabled should provide, on the one hand, compensation, and on the other hand, vocational rehabilitation.

This realization on the part of the public of a need by the physically disabled for something more than workman's compensation was given expression in the form of legislation. The State of Massachusetts in 1918 became the first state to enact laws providing for the training of persons who, because of accidents in industry, were unable to continue their occupations. Other states followed, and at the time of the passage of the first national vocational rehabilitation law, twelve states had enacted legislation concerned with vocational rehabilitation. Most of the state laws conformed in whole or in part to a model vocational rehabilitation law proposed in 1918 by the Red Cross Institute for Crippled and Disabled Men, an institution rounded in New York City in 1917.

There were a number of federal legislative enactments which influenced the development of the vocational rehabilitation program although they were not directly or immediately aimed toward the ultimate Federal recognition of vocational rehabilitation and the passage of the act of 1920. The two most outstanding of these were the Smith-Hughes Act of 1917, which provided grants-in-aid to states in order to develop programs of vocational education; and the Smith-Sears Act of 1918 for the vocational rehabilitation of disabled soldiers, sailors and marines.

Smith-Fess Act of 1920
(Civilian Vocational Rehabilitation Act)

Three months after the passage of the Soldier Rehabilitation Act (Smith-Sears), a bill to provide for the promotion of the rehabilitation of persons disabled in industry or otherwise and their return to civilian employment was introduced in the Senate. This bill became a law on June 2, 1920. It provided for the vocational rehabilitation of all persons who are vocationally handicapped by reason of a physical defect or infirmity, whether congenital or acquired by injury, accident or disease, and who were or might be expected to become totally or partially incapacitated for a remunerative occupation.

Supplemental Acts to the Smith-Fess Law

The program as it existed under the Act of 1920 was considered to be a temporary one. The period from 1920 to 1924 was a trial period to allow the program to prove itself and attract public attention. The federal appropriations of $750,000 for the first year and $1,000,000 annually for the next three years was allotted to the states in the proportion which their population bore to the total population of the United States.

Federal Social Security Act

The next high point in the historical development of the program was in 1935, when the Federal Social Security Act was passed. This Act authorized an appropriation of $841,000 annually for vocational rehabilitation for the years 1936 and 1937. This amount was added to the appropriation made under the provisions of the Vocational Rehabilitation Act of 1920 and resulted in a total appropriation of $1,938,000 for vocational rehabilitation for each of the two years. This amount was again authorized in 1938 and was increased to $3,500,000 in 1939. Meanwhile, Congress in 1936 enacted the Randolph-Sheppard Law which extended preference to blind persons as operators of vending stands in Federal buildings.

Liberalized Interpretation of Existing Acts

The next important development in the program was not in the form of legislation but in the legal interpretation of existing acts. Historians believe this liberalism was an outgrowth of the New Deal and the Supreme Court's responsiveness to public demands in rulings involving social welfare.

Barden-La Follette Act of 1943

The next major development in the program, legislation, history-wise, was in 1943 when the Barden-La Follette or Vocational Rehabilitation Act of 1943 amended the Industrial Rehabilitation Act of 1920. This 1943 law authorized payments for physical restoration to reduce or eliminate disabilities and permitted service to the emotionally and mentally ill. Federal funds were made available for the costs of vocational rehabilitation of war-disabled civilians" and for the entire cost of state administration, including vocational guidance and placement. The law provided that other expenses were to be shared by the Federal government and the states on a dollar-for-dollar basis.

The Vocational Rehabilitation Act of 1954

The most recent development in the program was in 1954 when the Act of 1943 was amended and several significant additions were made. The 1954 law provided for Federal funds to be allocated to the states by formula for increased rehabilitation services and for new kinds of programs. The sums authorized increased from $30,000,000 beginning in fiscal year 1955 to $65,000,000 in fiscal year 1958, and thereafter as Congress should determine. These funds were available for grants to the states to assist them in meeting the costs of vocational rehabilitation services and for additional services not included in the 1943 Act as follows: (1) hospitalization necessary in connection with surgery or treatment without the time limitation provided in the 1943 law, (2) tools, equipment, initial stock, and supplies for rending stands; (3) the establishment of special rehabilitation facilities for disabled persons and workshops for the severely disabled, (4) small business enterprises for the severely handicapped under the state agency's management and supervision.

Three types of federal grants were authorized in the Vocational Rehabilitation Act of 1954. These were (1) grants to states to assist them in meeting the cost of the basic vocational rehabilitation program; (2) grants to the states to assist them in initiating extension and improvement projects; and (3) grants to the states and to public and other nonprofit organizations to meet part of the cost of research, demonstration, training and traineeships, and other special projects. The grants for basic rehabilitation services are allotted to the states by means of a special formula designed to provide a relatively higher percentage of federal funds for the less wealthy states. The federal share of these funds varies from a minimum of 50 percent of the cost of the program to a maximum of 70 percent. The grants for extension and improvement projects are allocated to the states on a population basis with three federal dollars matched by one state dollar. Grants for special projects are made by the Secretary of Health, Education and Welfare after receiving recommendations of the National Advisory Council on Vocational Rehabilitation provided in the Act.

The new law also specified some requirements to be included in state plans for vocational rehabilitation; it required the Secretary to develop cooperative programs with other agencies to facilitate placement; designated the state agency administering or supervising the administration of vocational education in the state, or a state agency primarily concerned with vocational rehabilitation as the administrative agency; and made provisions for a study of the needs of homebound physically handicapped individuals.

Review of the Past and Looking to the Future

Many years of service to the severely disabled and handicapped men and women of America have proved the worth of the State-Federal program for vocational rehabilitation. During the first 23 years of its existence, this program operated under limited legislative authority that made no specific provisions for physical restoration, which today is one of the vital services rendered to many thousands of Americans. In 1943, the program was strengthened by legislation providing for the present complete range of services, including medical, psychiatric, and hospital care. Prior to the enactment of that legislation, it was necessary for the program to "train around" the disabilities of its clients in order to fit them for work that they could do. Today the program can and does provide medical services to restore lost functions—and even to save human life.

The nearly 750,000 men and women in rehabilitation in 14 years after 1943 exceed, by a wide margin, the number provided with lesser services(210,000) during the preceding 23 years of the program's operation. Thus, the history of public vocational rehabilitation in the United States is divided into two major periods. Today we are looking forward to a third major period. That new period will begin when rehabilitation services are available to every American who needs them.

Philosophy and Principles

Every profession or discipline has a philosophy. It may or may not be written. It may be a simple expression of outlook and policy, but it is often highly developed, in some cases to the extent of having several related or divergent schools of thought. Although philosophy is usually pictured as preceding practice, it becomes modified by practice so that it is ever changing. This is especially true in new professions. Limitations may prevent or delay the implementation of philosophy.

Professional vocational rehabilitation, born in a turbulent period, is still in its infancy, and its philosophy has not crystallized. Because of this, it is difficult to identify some of the factors that usually are apparent in the history or practice of a profession. The evolution has been a rapid one, since the service is sensitive to the changing demands of the people, especially as these demands are translated into legislation.

The history of vocational rehabilitation shows an emerging pattern of changing ideas which society holds toward the handicapped individual- As in most institutions, emotional feelings preceded the intellectualization of a philosophy. This section of the paper is an attempt to formalize some of the feelings which society today has for individuals who suffer vocational handicaps because of circumstances beyond their control as these attitudes may be reflected in the policies of the service.

General Principles

1. Vocational Rehabilitation assumes that each individual has a right to be employed in a remunerative occupation.
2. The program of vocational rehabilitation is not a "money maintenance" program.
3. Properly trained rehabilitants are efficient workers—persons who have overcome vocational handicaps.
4. Rehabilitated persons are economic assets to society.
5. Vocational rehabilitation is a partner, not a competitor, with other agencies.
6. Rehabilitation counseling should be considered as a profession.

7. The concepts of rehabilitation are dynamic, not static.

8. Vocational rehabilitation is a State-Federal cooperative program.

9. The rehabilitation agency will conscientiously investigate and consider each reported case, and serve it on a "needs-of-the-client" basis.

10. The law does not change facts, and should not be used as an excuse to avoid "hard cases," nor yet ignored to extend unjustified accommodation.

11. On matters of case processing involving quantity or quality of production, the vocational rehabilitation service will not pit federal against state, state against state, state against counselor, counselor against counselor; counselor against client; or client against client.

12. Severely handicapped persons may be trained for most occupations.

13. Mentally handicapped persons can be rehabilitated.

14. Age is rapidly becoming an occupational handicap.

15. Self-care is not a justifiable goal for vocational rehabilitation.

Principles Relating to Services

1. Eligibility for services is partly based on the presence of a substantial employment handicap resulting from a physical or mental disability.

2. Eligibility for services is partly based upon whether there is a reasonable expectation that services can eliminate or lessen the severity of the handicap.

3. Payment for services by the agency is partly based on economic need.

4. Eligibility for services is partly based on requirements set by the individual states.

5. Every client should have the benefit of counsel and guidance.

6. When the plan is considered feasible, training should be offered to the client.

7. When necessary to render an individual employable, physical restoration services should be offered.

8. Each physical restoration case must be considered, not only on its individual merits, but on the basis of the authority, scope, and services of other agencies offering similar services.

9. Money may not be spent on physical restoration services until the case is "relatively stable or slowly progressive."

10. Maintenance and transportation can be justified as a necessary adjunct to the client's benefit from the other services.

11. Tools and equipment will be supplied in justifiable cases.

12. After vocational rehabilitation has made an individual into an employable member of society, there still remains the responsibility of placing the individual in a job which suits his qualifications.

13. After the client's handicap has been removed and he has been satisfactorily placed, he is no longer eligible for services unless something happens to cause an occupational handicap.

14. Some special disability cases can be given the best care, treatment or training in institutions.

15. Certain uniform rules of practice must be observed in state and local offices.

16. The state office should require enough, but not too many, reports from local offices.

Principles Relating to the Counselor's Personal Philosophy

1. The counselor must have a wholesome attitude toward the handicapped.

2. There is no place for rationalization in a counselor's philosophy.

3. The counselor should regard himself as a member of a profession.

4. The counselor must hold an enlightened attitude toward the mentally handicapped.

5. The counselor must regard the information on clients as confidential and this information must be given the same protection and ethical consideration as any other privileged communication.

6. The Vocational Rehabilitation Counselor must see in his client some prospect of future vocational usefulness.

7. The counselor must be able to adjust himself to the community in which he works.

❦

CHAPTER EIGHT

KEYS TO THE REHABILITATION AND PLACEMENT OF THE MENTALLY ILL

James S. Peters, II, Ph.D.
Director, Bureau of Vocational Rehabilitation
Connecticut State Department of Education
and
Cyrus G. Flanders, Technician
Connecticut State Employment Service

Would you employ a former inmate of a mental hospital if the doctors said that he is now "in full remission?" Would you be afraid to work with such a person?

If so you would be in the majority. The tragedy of it is that your fears would be groundless. A person in full remission is fully cured and no more in danger of becoming mentally ill again than you or I are of becoming a patient in an institution.

Fear is the biggest road block in the way of employment for the mentally handicapped.

Just the other day, Mrs. Ethelind Collins, counselor in the Hartford office, was telling us that an employer had called the placement interviewer, and said "I'm sorry that I couldn't hire Anna. She was just what you said she was, and just what I wanted, but I have learned that she was in a mental hospital six years ago and I don't dare take a chance on her."

Anna had been in a mental hospital, but was discharged as fully cured, or "in full remission." She had been successfully employed ever since.

On the same day that Mrs. Collins heard about Anna's failure to land a job she was visited by a woman who had been advised to enter a mental hospital for an extended stay. Her question was, "Who will hire me if I have been in a hospital for three months?" She was not willing to undergo the

Published in the Monthly Bulletin, September 1958

45

treatment that would cure her because of her fear that she would not be hired after she was well again!

Two years ago, Thomas I. Shea, Director of the Connecticut State Employment Service, decided to do something about this fear. "Our counselors must be better informed about the patients who come out of mental hospitals if we are to talk convincingly with employers about those who are ready to work again," he said.

Training Sessions

With the cooperation of David K. Boynick, Assistant to the Commissioner of the State Mental Health Department and of Dr. John M. Bellis, Coordinator of Research and Training in that Department, a series of three in-service-training meetings were arranged, to be held at the three State mental hospitals. The first was held at Fairfield State Hospital, Newtown, the second at the Connecticut State Hospital, Middletown and the third at Norwich State Hospital. Present, in addition to personnel from the hospital and the Employment Service, were representatives of the Bureau of Vocational Rehabilitation, the Veterans Administration, the Veterans employment Service, and the Board of Education of the Blind. The Employment Service cooperates very closely with all of those Agencies in the rehabilitation and placement of all handicapped workers. When any of these Agencies gives trainings for their staff members, representatives of the other Agencies are invited.

The principal benefit that the Employment Service hoped to get from these meetings was that their counselors and selective placement interviewers and veterans' employment representatives would have a better understanding of the mentally ill so that they could serve employers more adequately, and, at the same time, meet their responsibilities to those mentally handicapped workers who are actually employable. Furthermore, there was a need for the employment Service to understand the problems confronting the Hospitals, and conversely, for the Hospitals to know more about the Employment Service than they did. Lines of communication were in need of clearing so that each knew what kind of information the other needed and could be aware of the need to give it promptly and completely.

"Is a victim of schizophrenia employable, and if so, under what conditions?" "How about the psychopathic personality? Can he be hired safely? If so, what working conditions should be avoided?" "When, if ever, can the person who has suffered from manic-depressive psychosis be employed?" These were some of the questions the Employment Service hoped to find the answers to. Without some authoritative information to these and other questions, no counselor or selective placement interviewer would dare to refer a mentally handicapped worker, no matter how well he seemed to fit the employer's requirements. The Employment Service can never forget that it has a responsibility to serve the employer as well as the worker. Failure to remember this can quickly "kill the goose that lays the golden egg."

The Rehabilitation Process

The agenda provided for talks by members of the medical staff at the hospitals who provided the background that made it possible to give the answers to these questions. They told also of the follow-up work that is being done at clinics in some of the communities throughout the State. Social workers told of the part that they play in the rehabilitation process. Physical therapists showed their patients busily at work in the laundry, in the bakery and at wood working, at weaving and painting.

One patient told of her experiences before she came to the hospital, the two years she had spent there, the new joy she was training for through the help of the Bureau of Vocational Rehabilitation, and of her impending departure to work for an employer who had already made arrangements to hire her.

The Bureau of Vocational Rehabilitation has assigned trained counselors to each of the three hospitals. They spoke of the part they play as members of the rehabilitation team. It was interesting to learn that as soon as the doctors decide that the patient is ready for work, they sit down with the occupational therapists, the social workers, the rehabilitation counselor and other team members to discuss the patient's future. Each gives complete information so that all may have a picture to guide them in their efforts to assist the patient. In some cases, the latter is present. If the patient needs a prosthetic appliance, the Bureau of Vocational Rehabilitation counselor arranges to furnish it for him. If it is decided that he needs training in a new type of work, the counselor arranges for instruction or on-the-job training, buys or rents the necessary equipment, pays for room and board, or arranges for it through the Welfare Department in the area where the patient is to study, and works closely with the Employment Service to locate a job opportunity for him when his training is finished and the Hospital gives the O.K. for his release.

Selective Placement Counts

A representative of the Employment Service described the counseling and selective placement services that are available, and stressed the fact that the referral interviewer must have the necessary information regarding the worker to enable him to properly carry out the function of the Employment Service which is to "match the man and the job." "If we attempt to make placements on sympathy alone, we will soon lose the employer's business." he said. He also gave some helpful information as to the best time to send or bring the patient into the local office, whom to contact there, and the type of information that the Employment Service must have.

The lively question period that followed each meeting was proof that the sessions were profitable. Everyone who attended was deeply impressed with the genuine interest there is in the problems of the mentally handicapped and the spirit of cooperation that exists between all the agencies who try to solve them. Furthermore, each learned much about the services given by the other, and how to use those services to better advantage.

The result has been better service to the mentally ill all the way through the rehabilitation process to employment in a job and adjustment on it.

Cooperation is a two way street. We have seen how the mentally ill have been rehabilitated after they have reached the hospital. How does the patient get to the doctor in the first place? There are many ways, of course, but one way is for the counselor in the Employment Service to recognize the worker's need for treatment when he comes in looking for a job. If he is incoherent in his talk or rambles, or has a marked suspicion of others, or shows unusual irritability, or any of the other symptoms, the alert counselor considers that he may need some professional assistance. He will attempt to make an appointment for him with the Bureau of Vocational Rehabilitation counselor who is due to spend several hours in the Employment Service Office within a few days. Cooperative arrangements have been made between the Directors of the Employment Service and the Bureau of Vocational Rehabilitation so that Bureau counselors visit each of the twenty local offices of the Employment Service once a week, or in a few cases, once in two weeks.

Once the BVR counselor agrees that the worker needs help, the doctors are called in for diagnosis and the patient receives needed treatment, including hospital treatment, if necessary. Whatever services he needs for complete rehabilitation are given to him. When he is ready for employment, he is referred back to the Employment Service for placement.

"Half-Way House"

One of the most heartening developments in the rehabilitation of the mentally ill is the experiment at Undercliff Hospital, Meriden, formerly a hospital for the tubercular, but now the half way house for men and women who have been victim of severe mental illness. Into this friendly institution come patients who have spent months and in some cases years in the other mental institutions. Here, for the first time, they are to experience a measure of freedom. There are no locks on the doors. Occasionally, even this limited amount of freedom is too much for the patient to take and he is returned to the more regimented routine to which he has been accustomed.

Dr. DeLavergne says, "The philosophy of treatment here is based on the fact that by providing opportunity for dignity, freedom, and responsibility, the patient will be better prepared to re-enter community living." Thus, Undercliff serves as the half-way house back to normal living. The patient lives there while he makes his first attempts to get out into a community again, to be trained there, to work there. The results of the experiment have been encouraging.

Let's take a look at one case to see what actually happened to Mrs. X. There isn't enough space in an article of this kind to do more than sketch an outline of what went on during her rehabilitation. We'll have to leave it to you to imagine Mrs. X's feelings as she was helped to work her way back into the community again.

The Case of Mrs. X

Mrs. X was transferred to the Undercliff Hospital on extended visit from Fairfield State Hospital, Newtown, Connecticut. (A person on "extended visit" can be returned to Fairfield Hospital or Middletown or Norwich at any time within a year, without commitment procedures). Her diagnosis was schizophrenic reaction, paranoid type in remission. Since she had made considerable progress at Fairfield, the medical team there felt that she could probably profit from the more extensive rehabilitation services provided by Undercliff.

Upon arrival at Undercliff, Mrs. X was evaluated as to her potential social, emotional, and vocational progress by the rehabilitation team. This team is composed of Doctors Paul M. DeLavergne, Walter Lohrman and L.E. Thompson; Psychiatrists, Theodore Pausig and Anselem Shurgast; Social Worker, Mrs. Mildred Puglisi; Nurse, Mrs. Barbara Fenn; and rehabilitation counselors, Bruce Cole and Robert Payne of the Bureau of Rehabilitation. It was found that her previous vocational experience was that of a school teacher in Canada. She had also done some clerical work both in Canada and in the United States. She is a very attractive, neat appearing person of approximately forty-five years of age. She was born and reared in Canada. After marriage, she came to this country and settled in a small Connecticut town. Shortly after building a home, she and her husband were divorced and she became pre-occupied with religion. Such preoccupation led to some bizarre behavior, which resulted in a superficial attempt at suicide. She was committed to Fairfield where she spent nearly two years.

Tests and Interests Considered

The Rehabilitation team at Undercliff recommended that the patient be seen frequently by the rehabilitation counselor, Mr. Payne. Mr. Payne administered a battery of psychological tests which consisted of an intelligence test, a vocational interest inventory, a personality inventory and several aptitude tests. From the test results, and background of work experience, coupled with the client's own expressed interest, it was decided that the clerical area should be explored for training and eventual job placement. The patient felt that school teaching would aggravate her emotional condition, should she return to it. Through the Bureau of Vocational Rehabilitation services, which includes financial support, the patient enrolled in and completed an eleven month course in book-keeping and clerical work at Laurel Business College in Meriden. Her grades were above average and she made a good adjustment at the school while continuing to live in the hospital.

Prior to the completion of her training, Mrs. X was encouraged by the counselor to register at the Meriden Office of the Connecticut State Employment Service. She was interviewed and counseled for possible job placement by Charles Reardon, Counselor and Selective Placement Interviewer.

Upon graduation, Mrs. X was employed by the Laurel Business School for approximately one month. Through the combined efforts of Mr. Payne and Mr. Reardon, Mrs. X was placed in a job with a public accountant where her work was very satisfactory. At the end of four months her job terminated. She registered with the employment service. After a short period of unemployment, a position was secured for her in the business office of a community hospital where she has been an excellent employee for over a year. She is now well adjusted in every way and has moved out of the half-way house.

The fact that Mrs. X was rehabilitated and placed and is back in the community again, even though her case would have been labeled hopeless only a few years ago, is cause for gratification, but not for complacency. It is an indication of progress made and a hopeful sign that more progress may come.

CHAPTER EIGHT

It will come, too, if all the agencies and associations continue to cooperate, and to learn, to improve their methods, and if ways can be found to dissipate the fear that stops the employer from hiring a man who is "in full remission."

ALCOHOLISM AND VOCATIONAL REHABILITATION

James S. Peters, II, Ph.D.
Director, Bureau of Vocational Rehabilitation
Connecticut State Department of Education

The vocational rehabilitation of the "problem drinker," or rather still, the "drinker with problems," presents a real challenge to rehabilitation workers. After 30-odd years of legal and professional status we are still baffled by the degree and complexity of the alcoholic problem, so much so until we have been, to a greater or lesser extent, overwhelmed by it. In meeting the problem state agencies of vocational rehabilitation are notorious for their inaction rather than action.

Vocational rehabilitation of the physically and mentally handicapped is a community program supported by both state and federal funds. Through the Office of Vocational Rehabilitation, Department of Health, Education and Welfare, funds are made available by the Congress to states on a matching basis. Amendments to the Vocational Rehabilitation Act, better known as The Vocational Rehabilitation Act of 1954, greatly increased funds for state and federal programs and, conversely, increased the size and scope of the program.

For example, in the United States in fiscal 1955, federal and state funds spent for administration, counseling, and case services totaled $38,636,578. The number of cases rehabilitated in that same fiscal year was 57,981.

In fiscal 1958, three years later, the federal and state funds spent totaled $67,517,000, an increase of 75% over 1955. Vocationally rehabilitated cases numbered 74,320, an increase of 28%. This small percentage

A paper delivered at the Northeast States' Conference on Alcoholism, New Haven Motor Inn, New Haven, Connecticut, Tuesday, May 19, 1959, sponsored by Conn. Commission of Alcoholism with grant from National Institute of Mental Health.

increase in rehabilitated cases compared with percent of state and federal funds allocated is attributed to several causes, a major one being severe personality problems in which is included a number of clients under the syndrome alcoholism.

In a recent study of problems of status 6 cases (ready for employment) in our agency by the Office of Vocational Rehabilitation and our staff, an attempt was made to validate or disprove five basic assumptions as to why Status 6 continues to increase.

They are as follows:

> 1. The recession has caused a drastic reduction in placement opportunities and rehabilitations and an increase in Status 6 cases.
>
> 2. Status 6 cases represent the more difficult cases because of the composition of this group of cases, which contains:
>> a. the more severely disabled—e.g., severe paralytics, severe mental illness cases, markedly limited mental retardates, grand real epileptics and those with multiple disabilities,
>>
>> b. more clients likely to have personality problems which would adversely affect placement, e.g., the alcoholics,
>>
>> c. and clients whose major impairment coupled with older age make placement more difficult.
>
> 3. Most of these cases are counseling, guidance, and placement only cases.
>
> 4. The vocational objective selected was not suitable in terms of the clients functional limitations, ability to acquire the necessary skills, and opportunity for placement in the objective selected in a given community.
>
> 5. These cases had not been accorded as much attention as cases in other statuses.

Procedure Used in the Study

Our agency selected every fourth case in the Status 6 caseload in each district office using a cutoff date, December 31, 1958. There were 271 cases in the Status 6 caseload in the Hartford District Office, as of that date. Selection of every fourth case would have produced a sample of 67 cases. However, one case classified in Status 6 subsequent to December 31, 1958, was excluded from the sample because of the fact, leaving a selected sample of 66 cases.

There were 233 cases in the Status 6 caseload in the Bridgeport District Office, as of the cutoff date. Selection of every fourth case would have produced a sample of 58 cases. However, eight cases had to be excluded from the initial selection in that office because they had been classified in Status 6 somewhat later than the cutoff date agreed upon. In order to complete the sample and make it as nearly comparable to the Hartford sample as possible, six cases were chosen at random from the remainder of the Status 6 case sample the office had available at the time the study was conducted.

This resulted in the selection of a total of 122 cases, 66 cases from the Hartford District Office and 56 cases from the Bridgeport District Office. These cases comprised 24% of the Status 6 caseload in the agency.

FINDINGS OF STUDY
Relation of Study Findings to Basic Assumptions

State agency personnel feel the recession has caused a reduction in placement opportunities and rehabilitations, and that this situation has contributed to the increase in the agency's Status 6 caseload. The usual progression of case movement from Status 6, ready for employment, is into Status 7, in employment, (to determine whether or not the vocational objective selected is suitable) and then into Status 12, closed, rehabilitated-(Cases are closed, rehabilitated, after it has been determined, through a period of observation by the counselor, that the vocational objective, selected jointly by the counselor and the client, is suitable.)

The March 1959 issue of "The Labor Market and Employment Security," page 77, contains a table, "Non-agricultural Placements by Major Occupational Group, 1958," which shows the percentage changes in placements from calendar 1957 through calendar 1958, made by the Employment Service in Connecticut, in the following occupational groups:

a. Professional and managerial	– 1.6%
Clerical and Sales	– 5.4%
Service	–11.5%
Skilled	+18.5%
Semiskilled	–12.7%
Unskilled and Other	–19.9%

b. In this same publication on page 78, there is a table showing how placements, in the industries listed, declined, as follows, between calendar 1957 and calendar 1958:

Construction	−12.4%
Manufacturing	−15.9%
Wholesale and Retail Trade	− 7.6%
Service (total)	− 7.4%

"Area Labor Market Trends," also published by the U.S. Department of Labor, classifies an area as meeting the requirements for designation as an 'area of substantial labor surplus' or 'area of substantial unemployment,' if the ratio of unemployment to the total labor force is 6% or higher. In Connecticut the following cities and towns were so designated as of December 31, 1958: Bridgeport, New Britain, New Haven, Waterbury, Ansonia, Bristol, Danbury, Danielson, Meriden, Middletown, Norwich, Thompsonville, Torrington and Willimantic. These data confirm the assumption made by State agency personnel that the recession has caused a reduction in placement opportunities which has in turn contributed to the increase in the agency's Status 6 caseload.

    2. The assumption that the Status 6 caseload contains many of the more difficult cases served by the agency appears to have some foundation.

        a. Severe paralytics, mental illness cases of psychoses in remission and severe anxiety states, mental retardates with intelligence quotients in the 50's and low 60's, grand real epileptics and clients with severely handicapping multiple disabilities would be included in the more severe disability groups served by any general agency. There were 31 such cases in the Hartford District Office sample. This number constituted 47% of the Status 6 caseload in that office. In the Bridgeport District Office sample there were 23 such cases, constituting 41% of the Status 6 caseload.

        b, Those clients likely to have personality problems which would affect their placement would be individuals who had. suffered a severe mental illness, the markedly mentally retarded, grand real epileptics, and tuberculosis cases. The last group is included because so many of the Status 6 cases reviewed, in *which tuberculosis was the major impairment, revealed alcoholism was also a formidable obstacle to rehabilitation. The 26 cases in these four* groups in the Hartford District Office comprise 39% of the Status 6 caseload, and the 18 cases in the Bridgeport District Office constitute 32% of their caseload. This indicates there is some basis for the assumption that many clients among the Status

6 cases do have personality problems which make placement difficult, but they do not constitute the bulk of the caseload.

c. Considering clients 40 years of age and over as the older age group, there appears to be foundation for the assumption that the Status 6 caseload contains many clients whose major impairment coupled with older age, makes placement in employment, and rehabilitation, more difficult. There were 37 such cases (56%) of the caseload in the Hartford District Office and 27 cases (48%) in the Bridgeport District Office caseload. Since these cases comprised more than one-half of the caseload in one office and very close to half Of the caseload in the other office surveyed, the assumption does not appear unwarranted.

3. There also appears to be a sound basis for assuming that most of the cases in the Status 6 caseload are counseling, guidance, and placement only cases, since two cases out of every three reviewed received only this service. There were 81 cases comprising 66% of the total agency caseload, with 46 out of the 66 cases sampled in the Hartford District Office and 35 of the 56 cases sampled in the Bridgeport District Office. Whether or not all of these cases should have been counseling, guidance, and placement only cases, is a question that will be touched upon a little later.

4. Eighteen cases, or 32% of the sample, in the Bridgeport District Office were cases in which the vocational objective did not appear to be suitable in terms of the client's functional limitations, ability to acquire the necessary skills, and opportunity for placement in a given community. There were 15 cases, or 22%, in the Hartford District Office sample in which the selection of vocational objective did not appear suitable.

5. It appears that the longer a case remains in Status 6, the less likely it is that it will receive attention, particularly after it has been in this status three months or more.

Summary

It appears that some of the assumptions frequently made as to why the Status 6 caseload in the Connecticut Bureau of Vocational Rehabilitation is so large and continues to grow are well-founded, whereas others do not tend to be as firmly supported by the findings of the study. There is evidence that the recession has caused a reduction in placement opportunities and contributed to the agency's Status 6 caseload. Substantial unemployment reduces the number of opportunities to move clients from

Status 6, ready for employment, into Status 7, in employment; or from Status 6 directly into Status 12, closed, rehabilitated.

There is fairly substantial evidence to support the contention that a sizable portion of the Status 6 caseload contains many clients whose major impairment coupled with older age makes placement difficult, that a high percentage of Status 6 cases are counseling, guidance, and placement only cases, and that the longer a case remains in Status 6, the less likely it is to receive attention, particularly after it has been in this status for three months or more.

There is some basis for the assumption that clients with personality problems are more difficult to place in employment and to rehabilitate than clients who do not have such problems, but such cases do not constitute the bulk of the Status 6 caseload.

There were enough cases in each district office in which the vocational objective did not appear to be suitable in terms of the clients' functional limitations, ability to acquire the necessary skills, and opportunity for placement in a given community, to indicate that considerably closer attention should be accorded the selection of a suitable vocational objective by the counselors.

The impact of the recession, the severity of the disabilities in the various groups comprising the Status 6 caseload, the frequency with which they appear, and the sizable percentage of older disabled clients are factors which the agency should take into consideration in its program plans, but they are not factors over which the agency can exercise very much control.

Our study of Status 6 cases clearly points out that our major concern for the moment is in the rehabilitation of the tubercular alcoholic. One reason for this is due to our experience with this type of patient through a three-year extension and improvement project grant from the Office of Vocational Rehabilitation. Some $45 to $50,000 were matched with federal funds which enabled us to employ three additional rehabilitation counselors to devote full time to work with patients in all of our state mental and tuberculosis hospitals.

During the past few years the tuberculosis in remission cases has constituted about 25% of our caseload. In spite of the success which we have had with this disabled group on the whole, we can say without fear of impunity or criticism that we have had little success with the patient whose tubercular condition was associated with alcohol. Our staff feels that the "most valuable result obtained from our experience with the tuberculous alcoholic in the state sanatoriums was the revelation of the need for education among staff on the nature of the problems of alcoholism before rehabilitation in such a setting is attempted."[1]

At the risk of sounding naive, most program or educational lag where the handicapped is concerned can be traced to prejudice. The alcoholic is a "socially handicapped" member of society like the psychopath, the delinquent, the unmarried mother, etc., even though there are fairly well defined psychological, physiological and chemical bases for the malady. Nevertheless, he has to suffer the rejection, isolation and frequently, deprivation which any despised minority must face. Prejudice toward the-handicapped is bad enough, but when the condition is tinted with experiences having overtones of "immorality and sin," even the most enthusiastic professional worker has a tendency to develop blind spots in his attempts to evaluate and plan a program with the client. It is this intolerance for ambiguity by workers from a predominate middle-class culture, I am afraid, which keeps a potential "space program" for the alcoholic from getting little farther than the "count down."

Prejudice toward handicapped persons with their open or hidden rejection by the non-handicapped occurs at every socioeconomic level of our society. It is evident in the social, educational, and vocational discriminations which hamper disabled persons. Gellman (2) in a recent article says:

> In the last analysis, it is the individuals who exhibit prejudice and reject disabled persons. It is the "I" rather than the "he" who commits discriminatory actions.
>
> The roots of prejudice come to fruition in the attitude and behavior of a non-handicapped John Doe toward a handicapped Richard Roe.
>
> Prejudice toward the disabled is seldom the result of chance factors. It is rooted in the prior life experience of the non-handicapped, who use prejudice to satisfy personal or social needs such as conformity to social custom, maintenance of self-esteem, enhancement of status, alleviation of personal fears, or increased self-respect.

Although, traditionally, rehabilitation agencies have experienced difficulty in attempting to rehabilitate the alcoholic, I do want to call to your attention two promising projects currently under way, from which we might learn more about working with this group. The first, a demonstration project, has been developed by the Arkansas Vocational Rehabilitation Service, Little Rock; the second, a research project, has been designed by the Salvation Army, Harbor Lights Center, Chicago, Illinois, in cooperation with Leroy N. Vernon and Associates.

In July 1957, sufficient funds were made available to the Arkansas Vocational Rehabilitation Service to enable the program to expand into areas which had hitherto been left unexplored because of the lack of funds for personnel and services. One of these areas is that of the alcoholic. In August 1957, a rehabilitation counselor was employed to work entirely with the alcoholic- He is a former alcoholic and is able to understand the problems of the group thoroughly and sympathetically- To date he has, with the cooperation of AA groups, understanding businessmen, and interested individuals, been able to help a great many of these unfortunate persons return to employment or train for employment they can follow.

A recent letter from a young woman who has been trained as a practical nurse through this program tells something of what it means to such a person to have a helping hand in the form of rehabilitation service:

> If this letter seems a little unusual to you, I will try to make it a little more understandable for you by telling you first my name is Jane Doe, and I am an alcoholic; also that I have just completed a year's schooling with the help of the Arkansas Vocational Rehabilitation Service. My reason for the letter is to offer in some small way my thanks because I am so grateful for the help I have received...
> January 16, 1958, was the last time I have had to have a drink. On that day I made my first contact with Alcoholics Anonymous which, thank God, gave me a second chance that very few people get to start a new life at my age. It was through this organization that I met my wonderful friend, the Rehabilitation Counselor for Alcoholics who, after hearing my story and believing in me, offered me a chance to become able to learn a way to be of some use to myself and other people, which no other person had ever done. I chose the one thing I had wanted to do all my life—nursing."

With a grant of $4,600 from the State of Illinois to the Salvation Army, Harbor Lights Center, Chicago, a research project on screening applicants was designed and put into operation. The Chicago Harbor Lights Center operates a religious and social program for the recovery and rehabilitation of the skid row alcoholic. This project has the approval of the Division of Alcoholism of the State Department of Welfare. Without going into detail I will merely cite its purpose:

To learn the characteristics of applicants who enter the rehabilitation program and attain some measure of progress toward rehabilitation as compared with those applicants who show little or no progress, so that such information may be useful in enabling the Center to achieve more in its rehabilitation efforts with its limited resources. It is assumed also, that this information will be useful to other rehabilitation programs which have similar intake problems.

The project is divided into four phases including a pilot study of 50 failures (AWOL's who deserted the program without leave) in contrast with the first 50 cases who remained in the program two weeks or longer. A total of 374 alcoholic subjects will be involved in the study. It is too early to predict outcomes for these two projects, but they are excellent examples of private and public efforts to get more objective or definitive information about the alcoholic from a rehabilitation angle. If more community agencies would follow this direction, it is my personal feeling that within the next five or six years there will be a greater degree of acceptance of the alcoholic for rehabilitation.

I would be remiss if I would not mention three rehabilitation research demonstration possibilities into alcoholism already proposed here in Connecticut. With adequate financial aid (local, state and/or federal) each, beyond a doubt, would add significantly to our knowledge as well as to our rehabilitated case load. They are:

1. A study of the vocational adjustment of two categories of problem drinkers and an analysis of the problems and potentialities of vocational counseling for these two categories. (A project designed by the Connecticut Commission on Alcoholism and submitted to the Office of Vocational Rehabilitation for a grant under Section 4 (a) (1) of the Vocational Rehabilitation Act, as amended.)

2. An experimental project for tuberculosis patients with drinking problems. (A project designed by Dr. Selden Bacon of the Connecticut Commission on Alcoholism with assistance from staff of the Bureau of Vocational Rehabilitation, Connecticut State Department of Education.)

3. An incomplete proposal for a project on "Rehabilitating the Chronic Drinker Through Environmental Manipulation." (Proposed by the Reverend Joseph Pouliot, Executive Director, Bridgeport Christian Union.)

Such projects as those named above, coupled with the excellent work already going on in the various clinics and the Compass Club operated by the Commission on Alcoholism would complement the present inadequate rehabilitative efforts among the alcoholics in Connecticut and the rest of New England. As our savant in such matters, Dr. Bacon (1, p.9) had said so well:

> It is important to the probably obvious point that no problem is going to be solved or even adjusted to in any adequate or satisfactory manner until the nature of the problem is well defined. If for example, drunkenness and drinking and alcoholism are indiscriminately regarded as a single problem then efforts to meet such a "problem" will be doomed to failure. The first step, then, is evaluation of the problem, recognition of misleading definitions and assumptions, and a tolerant, even humble attempt to locate and describe and analyze the matter under consideration.

It is my opinion that if rehabilitation workers and members of disciplines committed to alcoholism control and its eventual eradication would combine their forces for research and demonstration, a breakthrough could be accomplished within the foreseeable future. To this end we all should be dedicated.

Notes

1 Some problems in the rehabilitation of the tubercular alcoholic. Unpublished paper, Yale University Summer School of Alcoholic Studies, 1958.

References

1. Bacon, S. B., Alcoholism: Nature of the Problem and Alcoholism: Its Extent, Therapy and Prevention. Yale Center of Alcohol Studies, New Haven: 1956.

2. Gellman, W., Roots of Prejudice Against the Handicapped. Journal of Rehabilitation: Jan.-Feb. p. 25, 1959.

3. The Counselor, Vocational Rehabilitation Service, State Board of Education, Little Rock, Arkansas, March, 1959.

CHAPTER TEN

VISUAL REHABILITATION
OF THE AGING

James S. Peters, II, Ph.D.
Connecticut State Department of Education

In the White House Conference on Aging section on rehabilitation, a real attempt was made to keep in focus the broader concept of the term, i.e., independence.

The majority of the group, which ranged from interested lay delegates to professionals of all descriptions and hue, was committed to a medical, social, psychological, and economic philosophy of rehabilitation where the "team approach" to problems of the aging handicapped client is the principal model.

The definition of "rehabilitation" decided upon, after much discussion, was, and I quote:

"Rehabilitation is a philosophy and a set of skills and techniques directed toward helping the patient do as much as he can, as well as he can, for as long as he can. Such a definition takes into consideration not only the maintenance of current independence, but it also places an equally important emphasis upon the time element—for as long as he can."

Current interest in "independent living" legislation which is before the Congress, produced considerable discussion from those who would stick to the tradition of seeing rehabilitation as preparing the disabled for a vocation, to those who view rehabilitation in its broader concept, independence and/or some level of adjustment.

The prevailing idea of rehabilitation of the aging being everybody's business was questioned. Many present took exception to this notion. But even here, those who took exception inferred that although rehabilitation

A paper read at the 39th Annual Congress, New England Council of Optometrists, Statler-Hilton Hotel, Boston, Sunday, March 12, 1961.

of the aging may not be everybody's business, it certainly should be everybody's interest.

Exclusive of the direct physical medical implications during the "rehab" process, the discussions centered around the philosophy of rehabilitation as it applies to the dignity of our senior citizens in enabling them to lead lives as free of dependency upon others as possible.

The major areas for work group discussion were as follows:

A. Vocational Rehabilitation of Older Disabled People
B. Rehabilitation in the Practice of Medicine
C. Rehabilitation and Related Services within Institutions
D. Organization of Community Services to Meet the needs of the Disabled
E. Vision Loss among the Aging and the Aged
F. Hearing Loss among the Aging and the Aged

One can see from these that there was diversification of topics for work groups to discuss as well as people represented. In spite of pre-conference thinking, there was unanimity of opinion that the State-Federal vocational rehabilitation program should be broadened and more of our older age group included in its case load.

The delegates in the section on rehabilitation and, in particular, the work group concerned themselves with the following pertinent issues:

Goals of Rehabilitation
Extent of Disablement among Middle-Aged and Older Persons
Nature of Chronic Illnesses and Disability among the Aging
I will briefly discuss each.

Goals of Rehabilitation

Rehabilitation has the objective of providing services for the disabled individual that will help him to help himself to his fullest potentialities for whatever satisfactions he wants in life, and is able to attain. By providing help toward recovery of function and restoration of capacity, it is an important means for increasing independence, dignity, and self-respect among disabled persons in the later years. At one extreme, the maximum attainable goal may be progress from bed to wheelchair or an increased capacity for self-care. At the other extreme, it may be aimed at restoration to remunerative employment. The former is often designated as "rehabilitation for independent living;" the latter is designated as "vocational rehabilitation." It is with both types of rehabilitation that our section was concerned.

Extent of Disablement Among Middle-Aged and Older Persons

The most obvious facts about the American population are its expanding proportion of aging and aged people, and the increase in chronic disease or disabilities which becomes most apparent in the age groups 65 or over.

Fifty-two million people in the nation are age 45 or more. Over fifteen and one-half million or one-twelfth of the population are 65 or more. It is estimated that by 1980 some 68,400,000 of our population will be age 46 or more and that 24,500,000 of these people will be 65 years of age and over.

There is no single nationwide State-Federal program which provides rehabilitation services to severely disabled people to enable them to achieve independence in meeting the normal demands of daily living. However, most often the absence of such rehabilitation programs and services in our communities is the rule rather than the exception.

Nature of Chronic Illnesses and Disabilities among the Aging

Certain chronic illnesses and handicaps are more prevalent among aging persons than among younger people. These include diseases of the heart and other cardiovascular diseases, arthritis and rheumatism, cancer, orthopedic impairments, mental illness, loss of hearing, loss of vision and genitourinary diseases. No two people react in the same way to the same disease; these diseases, therefore, affect aging people and limit their activities to different degrees and in different ways.

We have experienced through our vocational rehabilitation programs a fair degree of success with the training and eventual job placement of visually handicapped clients. Recent evidence points toward vocational success of those fitted with optical aids. Time will not permit for more than one example.

Jennings of the University of North Carolina investigated the Blind Optical Aids Program of the North Carolina State Commission for the Blind. Of the 178 persons examined in the Optical Aids Clinic (Memorial Hospital, Chapel Hill) over a period of twenty-four examining days, 158 were fitted with optical aids. Of the 154 questionnaires sent to those who could be reached, there were 116 usable returns (75.3 percent). The ages of these 67 males and 49 females ranged from 10 to 62 with a mean of 30.5. There were 74 congenitally blind, 38 acquired blind, and 4 unknown. Educational level ranged from two years to 19 years of school completed, with a mean of 10.2.

The use of optical aids, the questionnaire responses indicate, improved the ability of both the congenitally and acquired blind in four of the social and cultural items, such as reading newspapers, books, personal mail, and looking up telephone numbers; a larger percentage of the acquired blind, however, received such benefit. In the other eight social-cultural items, such as seeing television, seeing the movies, walking about, seeing scenery while riding in a car, recognizing friends, shopping, doing homework, and doing their personal grooming, the use of optical aids yielded no improvement in either group.

Regarding the economic items, such as: Has the use of optical aids helped you to get a job, helped you to get a better job, helped you to increase your income, and helped you to perform your job with greater ease, it was found that the acquired blind had received more economic benefits from the use of optical aids. Concerning attitudes, the data reveal a larger percentage of the congenitally blind as pleased with their optical aids and wearing them in public places.

The males in grades 9 through 12 and the females in grades 1 through 8 received the most social-cultural and economic benefits. The males had a better attitude toward optical aids and the optical aids program than did the females. It was interesting to note that optical aids had helped the males only in the reading items, while they had helped the females in the reading items plus two other social-cultural items, namely in seeing television and recognizing friends.

If older persons who are visually handicapped were provided modern rehabilitation services, many could once again learn to live their lives in independence and with greater respect and dignity. Some could even return to work. others could be brought to conditions of independent living or self-care. In either case, the benefits from rehabilitation services would extend not only to the disabled persons alone, but to their families and to society as a whole. For those who returned to work, lost wages would be restored, industry would regain needed labor skills, and there would be new purchasing power and tax revenues in our sagging economy. For those who were freed from constant attendance or dependency, institutional and welfare costs would often be decreased.

ॐ

CHAPTER ELEVEN

REHABILITATION FOR THE SOCIALLY HANDICAPPED: EMPLOYMENT INDEPENDENCE

**James S. Peters, II, Ph.D.
Division of Vocational Rehabilitation
Connecticut State Department Education**

The restoration of employable welfare clients to self-support through a work training process is a laudable, humanitarian undertaking by the State of Connecticut. Governor John Dempsey and the Commissioners of Welfare, Health, Mental Health, and Education are to be congratulated for taking on such a bold program cooperatively. Those of us who have been involved with Commissioner Shapiro and his staff in conceptualizing the project have found the experience exciting as well as challenging.

As State Director of our Vocational Rehabilitation Program I have long questioned the exclusion of the socially handicapped from our program. If public welfare recipients are able-bodied, i.e., free from disease and physical and/or mental conditions of an aggravating nature, they should be entitled to vocational rehabilitation. A social handicap is just as embarrassing, self-effacing, self-rejecting and economically wasteful as a physical or mental handicap.

Public welfare organizations carry a host of indigents on their roles who have never had a decent opportunity to experience work of a meaningful nature due to their inability to initiate a program of satisfactory work opportunity. You may say such people are lazy, stupid, or just plain lacking in motivation, but we have seen social workers and rehabilitation counselors working as a team change such individuals into productive workers. A special Office of Vocational Rehabilitation project was estab-

---

A talk delivered at the Institute on Work Training for Welfare Clients, Department of Public Welfare, Hartford, Connecticut, August 16, 1962.

67

lished in Dade County, Florida, entitled "Hope" and designed to rehabilitate fathers in families receiving Aid to Dependent Children as a prototype project in this area of work. Last year, our own Bureau of Vocational Rehabilitation and the Department of Public Welfare undertook a similar project and experienced some degree of success for a short period of about eight months.

The big push for the vocational rehabilitation of welfare clients has come from the Public Welfare Amendments of 1962, House of Representatives Report No. 2006, and No. 10606 of the Senate. In these amendments, and especially through Title I, Part A, provisions are made to prevent or reduce dependency through state and federal efforts. This is purely and simply the rehabilitation philosophy.

Some of the more definitive aspects of rehabilitation may be gleaned from its philosophy and definitions. W. Scott Allan, in his book on the *Community and Rehabilitation* sets forth the philosophy of rehabilitation, thusly:

> the basic concern of rehabilitation is not professions or disciplines, not facilities or techniques, not agencies or programs, but people. Human beings do not live as isolated individuals, neither do they suffer in isolation. This means that restoration of the handicapped person to a fuller existence, a greater opportunity, does not happen by chance but neither is it the particular province of any one profession or group. It is rather the responsibility of the community it calls for community planning, action and support.

Howard Rusk, M.D., a well-known leader in the rehabilitation movement, says:

> Rehabilitation is not just splints, crutch walking, and the like. It has to meet the total needs of the individual; those needs are physical, emotional, social, and vocational, and at any time you miss a cog in the link then your morbidity goes up, and also your mortality; not the mortality of death but the mortality of something that is sometimes more than death, mortality of living a life of indignity, of dependency and depression.

CHAPTER ELEVEN

Definitions of Rehabilitation

Rehabilitation is an organized and systematic process by which the physical, mental, and vocational powers of the handicapped individual are improved to the point where he can compete with equal opportunity with the so-called non-handicapped. The process should start at the time of illness or accident and extend to the time of maximum physical, emotional, social and economic adjustment.

—Selected Readings on Rehabilitation,
IllinoisPublic Aid Convission, 1955

Rehabilitation is the restoration of the handicapped to the fullest physical, mental, social, vocational, and economic usefulness of which they are capable.

—National Council on Rehabilitation
Symposium on the Process of
Rehabilitation

Rehabilitation is making a person aware of his potential and then providing him with the means of attaining that potential.

—Scott Allan
Rehabilitation—A Community Challenge

Rehabilitation is whatever is necessary to get handicapped people from where they are to where they ought to be in view of their potential.

—Mary E. Switzer
Director Office of Vocational Rehabilitation

The above and selected research and demonstration projects supported by OVR grants under 4(a)l of the Public Law 565 of 1954 have eventuated in administrative actions through rehabilitation programs to strengthen and improve services for public assistance applicants and recipients.

❦

CHAPTER TWELVE

VOCATIONAL REHABILITATION

James S. Peters, II, Ph.D.
Director, Bureau of Vocational Rehabilitation
Connecticut State Department of Education

Fellow Rotarians, visitors and guests, I deem it an honor as well as a pleasure to speak to you on a subject that is near and dear to my heart, not only because of my professional affiliation with it, but also due to my sincere interest in its cause and philosophy.

"Its cause is just," to borrow a trite phrase from the revolution makers; its philosophical undergirding is in the tradition of "true Americanism," to steal a phrase from the conservatives. The justness of the cause for the rehabilitation of the disabled or handicapped among us springs from our Judaic-Christian heritage which is an outgrowth of man's need to become his brother's keeper; his identification with suffering humanity; his desire for self emolument, perhaps, and/or his search for immortality. Nevertheless, the philosophical undergirding is something else, again.

I have stated that the thesis Vocational Rehabilitation is "true Americanism." This I believe to be a truism for vocational rehabilitation is "the process of restoring the handicapped individual to the fullest physical, mental, social, vocational, and economic usefulness of which he is capable." I wish to underscore "economic usefulness" for it is here where the rehabilitation movement fits into the best of democratic capitalism; it is in this area that we attempt to adhere to the proposition that every individual worth his salt, desires a job so that he might be a giver of bread rather than a receiver of alms; so that he might be a taxpayer rather than a welfare recipient of a welfare check. Then too, following in the best of Puritan dogma and Protestant ethics, every man should labor for God and for country.

A talk given at weekly meeting of Rotary Club, Hartford, Hotel Statler, Monday, April 6, 1964, and given at Rotary Club of West Hartford, Thursday, April 8, 1965.

In Vocational Rehabilitation, State Department of Education, through our state-wide system of local and district offices, we assist not only those capable of attaining full-time competitive employment in the labor market, but extend services to those persons who are only capable of part-time, sheltered, homebound, or self-employment.

The rehabilitation is concerned primarily with the handicapping problems resulting from disability and deals with those problems for which the individual lacks the necessary resources to minimize or remove and to make possible the greatest level of achievement within his capabilities. Vocational rehabilitation counseling is defined as a process which a physically or mentally disabled person undertakes in order to help him understand both his problems and his potentialities, and to carry through a program of adjustment and self improvement to the end that he will make the best possible vocational, personal, and social adjustment. In the main, it is a "human engineering" or "man salvage" job. It is conservatively estimated by Bureau of Labor statistics that for every $1.00 spent to rehabilitate a person, the state and federal governments receive $10.00 in taxes at the end of the first year.

The vocational rehabilitation counselor, also, offers rehabilitative services to those individuals whose disabling conditions occurred, prior to significant work experience (habilitation) as well as those engaged in gainful employment before acquiring a vocational handicap (rehabilitation). This is a public program for all citizens. Even the handicapped homemaker is eligible for vocational rehabilitation services. I think it is fitting to add here, that in the best of private enterprise tradition, all of our work with clients, the exception being that of counseling, is done on a contractual basis with hospitals, clinics, rehabilitation centers, practicing physicians, schools, colleges, business and industry, etc. We do not operate any competing centers, schools, etc. All of the work is farmed out on an established fee basis with administrative and state approval.

I would be remiss in my job of a public administrator if I failed to enlighten you relative to the state of affairs of our vocational rehabilitation program.

With the 1954 amendments to the federal Vocational Rehabilitation Act, services and federal money for the disabled were broadened considerably. It is estimated in the State of Connecticut, 3,600 disabled persons each year become in need of vocational rehabilitation services that are provided by the Bureau of Vocational Rehabilitation and the Board of Education of the Blind. In 1962 these two State agencies accepted for service about 45% of persons and rehabilitated back into employment about 26%. By comparison, Rhode Island accepted for services 100% of the total number of disabled persons becoming in need of the services provided by its vocational rehabilitation programs and rehabilitated back into employment about 64%.

In fiscal year 1961 (July 1, 1960 - June 30, 1961) $455,910 in Federal funds was available to Connecticut for its vocational rehabilitation programs. To receive this, State funds of $373,765 were required for matching; only $320,339 in State funds was appropriated. Therefore, $53,426 in Federal funds lapsed. In fiscal year 1962 (July 1, 1961 - June 30, 1962) $587,478 in Federal funds was available to Connecticut. To receive these, State funds of $543,386 were required; only $356,160 was appropriated. Therefore, $187,226 in Federal funds lapsed. In fiscal year 1963 (July 1 1962- June 30, 1963) $721,101 in Federal funds was available to Connecticut. To receive this, State funds of $721,101 were required; however, only $373,674 was appropriated. Therefore, in fiscal 1963, Federal funds in the amount of $347,427 went unused.

In 1956, Connecticut spent $553,249 for its vocational rehabilitation programs. In 1962, the amount spent was $711,486, an increase in the six-year period of 28%. By comparison, Rhode Island spent $206,562 in 1956 for its vocational rehabilitation program and $663,282 in 1962, an increase in the six-year period of 221%. Massachusetts spent $731,344 in 1956 for its vocational rehabilitation program and $2,283,057 in 1962, an increase in the six-year period of 220%.

Although vocational rehabilitation staff members in Connecticut are among the best prepared, professionally, in the country, the counseling staff up to 1965 has not increased in many years. In the Bureau of Vocational Rehabilitation in 1956 a total of 22 counselors was employed. As of June 30, 1962, the total number of counselors was still 22. During fiscal years 1959 and 1960 there were 21 counselors in the State. Actually, there has been no increase in number of counselors for the rehabilitation program in the past 10 years (1955-1965). In comparison, the Massachusetts Rehabilitation Commission had 20 counselors in 1956. As of September 30, 1962, there were 56 counselors on the staff. Rhode Island Division of Vocational Rehabilitation had 12 counselors in 1956. As of September 30, 1962, there were 29 counselors on the staff. Connecticut has one vocational counselor for approximately each 98,000 population. By comparison, Vermont has one vocational counselor for approximately each 49,600 population. Rhode Island has one counselor for approximately 48,600 population.

Between 1956 and 1962, the number of disabled persons rehabilitated through the Connecticut Bureau of vocational rehabilitation program decreased approximately 2% from 927 in 1956 to 907 in 1962. During this same period, the number of persons rehabilitated through the Rhode Island Division of Vocational Rehabilitation program increased 176% from 315 in 1956 to 871 in 1962; persons rehabilitated through the Massachusetts Rehabilitation Commission program increased 108% from 794 in 1956 to 1,661 in 1962; persons rehabilitated through the Maine Vocational Rehabilitation Division program increased 67% from 215 in 1956 to 360 in 1962; persons rehabilitated through the New Hampshire Vocational Rehabilitation Division program increased 80% from 105 in 1956 to 198 in 1962; persons rehabilitated through the Vermont Vocational Rehabilitation program increased 42% from 159 in 1956 to 226 in 1962.

The Federal Office of Vocational Rehabilitation made available to Connecticut this fiscal year $2,520 to use for in-service training of its staff. To receive this amount, the State had to match it with only $280. The Connecticut Department of Education has not used *State* funds to take advantage of this generous matching ratio. The Bureau Chief has been able to get other agencies to match these funds so that his staff could continue to receive excellent in-service training. These Federal in-service training funds are quickly taken advantage of by every other State.

The philosophy of the whole movement for rehabilitation of the handicapped was set forth in 1919 by Gerrard Harris (4) in what is probably the first book on rehabilitation published in this country.[1] The fundamental justification and aim of the work was held to be a "demand for social justice which no democracy can deny," the "avoidance of dependency." Thus, even at that time, the "right for independency" was the recognized basic humanitarian goal. That this right should not be limited to those injured in war was acknowledged. The plea was also made that rehabilitation is a necessary "conservation of human resources" (the Nation was particularly concerned at that time over the prospects of curtailed immigration due to the labor shortage in Europe). Then, as now, rehabilitation was described as a "wise business investment." Even today, we do not seem to be content with the humanitarian aspects of rehabilitation and feel compelled to shore up our argument in terms of the financial return of the dollar investment.

It is possible to state the guiding principles of rehabilitation as we conceive them in this country. The exclusion of other nations, many of which have their own fine programs, is a necessary one.[2] We in America have no prior claim to human decency, but it is expressed in ways unique to our own cultural heritage and beliefs as implemented by our material resources. Should it seem at times that we fail to achieve the theoretical ideal we set for ourselves, that, too, is understandable. Goals have functional value even when not fully achieved, perhaps especially then. The principles which are put forth below are just as valid for guides to the individual rehabilitation counselor in his direct work with his clients as they are to those responsible for program planning and administration.

Our fundamental belief is an abiding respect for the dignity of the individual. His inherent worth as a person is not to be obscured by cost accounting procedures whereby the substandard producer is written off as a poor investment. A human has intrinsic value and it is this which is paramount. The high position of man, in our esteem, derives from our religious and political beliefs. Economic evaluation of a human being is inappropriate. This concept is indeed basic to all others and must be accepted to understand the premises which follow:

1. We are committed to the conviction that the individual is the best judge of his own future. The concept of freedom to the individual is an essential element in creating a democratic society. The root of the rehabilitation process is reliance upon the client's right to self-determination and self-improvement. We accept the disabled person's right to make his own decisions, to work out his own problems, within the framework of a service which facilitates self-help. In rehabilitation, independence is both the goal and the means. Only occasionally, and then just to the extent of absolute necessity, is there any modification of the individual's freedom for self-direction.

2. We hold that equality of opportunity is a right. It follows that rehabilitation, whereby the ability of the individual is restored, is a right. Our goal in rehabilitation is to raise the individual to the highest possible level consistent with his own interests and potentialities. Minimal objectives are inconsistent not only with our theoretical objectives but also from the economic standpoint. We cannot countenance poverty, we are not appeased with subsistence, we are contented only when the full measure of opportunity for the individual is obtained. Restoration of opportunity is not a charity or a special privilege. It means every disabled man, woman and child possessing a remedial handicap to opportunity and not receiving such, is having his rights violated.

Unfortunately, there remains a very practical distinction between human or social rights and those which are implemented by law and facilities. In practice, we adhere to the realities operating today - restrictive though they may be. But this should not deter the formulation of principles even when they are operationally neglected for the lack of ways to implement them. Today in rehabilitation, we are surrounded by restrictions, restrictions in financing, eligibility requirements, staff, facilities, and techniques. But breadth of vision and the adoption of a firm philosophy is not beyond our control. This is our preparation for the challenge of tomorrow.

Having a fundamental philosophy to guide our thinking does not negate appreciation of its practical values in rehabilitation. We are still in the position of selling the program on the basis of an investment with concrete returns. There is nothing sordid about money, and there need be no hesitation in stating the fact that every dollar invested in rehabilitation is returned to our economy many times over. Indeed, such only illustrates the effectiveness of our procedures which restores human independency and permits the satisfaction of contribution. However, we must remember that this financial return is not the goal of rehabilitation but one of its many important results.

To predict the future, it is necessary to take our clues from the past. In examining the past, we can conclude that changes in the lot of the disabled depend primarily upon two factors: (1) improvement in the general economy and in technology, and (2) changes in attitudes of the public which bring about application of these improvements to the problems of the disabled. We have seen public attitudes change slowly and as a result there is much needless delay in implementing advancements after they become available. But as social attitudes are formulated, they are translated into social action employing technical and economic resources to the advantage of the handicapped. To answer the question of what we will do tomorrow for our disabled, we need only learn what can be done today - what is technically and economically feasible.

The most glaring inadequacy of our present rehabilitation program is the established fact that it reaches only a fraction of those who could profit from it. We can anticipate both horizontal and vertical expansion to include more of those now legally eligible as well as the disabled not now entitled to needed rehabilitative services.

Notes

[1] Another early text, Disabled Persons: Their Education and Rehabilitation by Oscar Sullivan and Kenneth A. Snortum (9), published in 1926, is of historical importance for establishment the terminology adhered to since in vocational rehabilitation.

[2] A general survey of the measures adopted in the various nations to facilitate the occupational re-establishment of disabled persons has been published by the International Labour Office (5).

🍂

CHAPTER THIRTEEN

THE 1965 VOCATIONAL REHABILITATION AMENDMENTS AND DEPRIVATION

James S. Peters, II, Ph.D.
Director, Division of Vocational Rehabilitation
Connecticut State Department of Education

The 1965 Vocational Rehabilitation Amendments of the vocational Rehabilitation Act is the first significant piece of legislation in the field since 1954. Those of us who are charged with the responsibility for implementing the amendment recognize the tremendous opportunity for broadening our state-federal program so that a greater number of deprived, neglected, and frequently forgotten people can be served.

In the June 1966 report of the Advisory Council on Public Welfare, President Lyndon B. Johnson is quoted as saying:

"Today, for the first time in our history we have the power to strike away the barriers to full participation in our society. Having the power, we have the duty."

Through the enactment of our 1965 amendments, the Congress has made it possible fort the federal-state aided VR programs to respond more effectively to some of the social and economic changes with which society must deal.

Enlightened and concerned workers in the Vocational Rehabilitation movement have worked diligently over the years for a program which would be broadened so that the socially, culturally, and educationally deprived could be eligible for our services. In December of 1963, I publicly

A talk given at the annual meeting of the National Rehabilitation Association, Wed., October 5, 1966, Denver, Colorado.
Talk also given at In-Service Training of DVR in cooperation with the Nationwide Insurance Company, Shoreham Hotel, October 27, 1966.

recommended amending the Vocational Rehabilitation Act so that such individuals could be included in our counselors' caseload This recommendation was made during the closing hours of a meeting of State Administrators of VR programs.

On Wednesday, June 2, 1965, Governor John Dempsey signed into law House Bill No. 3139, "An Act Establishing a Division of Vocational Rehabilitation within the State Department of Education." The Bill had received a favorable report by the Joint Committee on Education following a lengthy hearing. This Act went into effect on October 1, 1965, after recommendation by the Commissioner and approval by the State Board of Education.

With a greatly increased budget for vocational rehabilitation service during this biennium, the program has been broadened and improved considerably. The State's appropriation of nearly $718,100 the first year of the biennium (1965-1966), due to recent amendments, brought the Division to a 62.5% federal share basis, approximately $1,200,000. This will make a total of $1,918,100 available for the year. For fiscal 1966-1967, the State's appropriation is $904,000. The Federal appropriation for this period will be on a 75% federal matching basis. Therefore, it is estimated that approximately $2,347,000 will be available from the Vocational Rehabilitation Administration, Department of Health, Education, and Welfare, making the total allocation for Vocational Rehabilitation approximately $3,251,000 ($3,586,300 for biennium 1967-1968).

The new Vocational Rehabilitation Act Amendments (Public Law 89-333) passed by the Congress during its 1965 session have been instrumental in further strengthening the program of Vocational Rehabilitation. The new Grants-In-Aid Programs to workshops and rehabilitation facilities will enable the State of Connecticut to utilize more funds and facilities in our efforts to eradicate poverty and dependency.

We now have a total of 50 professional workers and 31 clerical workers, making a total of 81 workers in the Division.

In order to serve the disabled citizens of Connecticut to qualify for our program, the Division has recognized its services into an internal structure which can be geared most effectively to an external system with the State's regional concept as its model.

The new State Plan for Vocational Rehabilitation in Connecticut (1966), which was approved by the State Board of Education, gives a description of the program in keeping with Public Law 89-333 as promulgated by the Secretary of Health, Education, and Welfare. The Administrative and Services pattern follows:

1. *Designation of State Agency*

   a. The State Board of Education is given authority to maintain a Division of Vocational Rehabilitation which is designated as the sole agency to administer the vocational rehabilitation program, except for rehabilitation services to the blind.

   b. The Division of Vocational Rehabilitation is primarily concerned with the vocational and other rehabilitation of disabled individuals.

   c. The legal authority for such designation is contained in Public Act 91, enacted in 1965.

2. *Responsibility of State Agency*

All decisions affecting the eligibility of clients, the determination of rehabilitation potential, or the nature and scope of Vocational Rehabilitation Services to be provided, will be made by the Division of Vocational Rehabilitation and this responsibility will not be delegated to any other agency or individual not of the agency staff.

3. *Organization of the State Agency*

The Division of Vocational Rehabilitation, operating within the framework of the State Board of Education, and having equal status with other Divisions, is primarily concerned with vocational and other rehabilitation of disabled persons, and is responsible for the vocational rehabilitation program of the State of Connecticut, except for rehabilitation services for the blind.

   a. The Division of Vocational Rehabilitation maintains a central administrative office with bureaus, consultants, and advisory committee, as well as a system of district and local offices, strategically located throughout the State. There are five (5) district offices and thirteen (13) local offices. The central office through its bureaus, functions to provide direction, supervision, coordination, and overall fiscal management of the rehabilitation program. In addition, professional and technical information, research and consultative services are made available to district and local offices, and to private and public community agencies. The system of district and local offices functions to locate, investigate, evaluate, counsel, provide and supervise rehabilitation services to handicapped individuals found to be eligible for needed services. Local offices, under the supervision of a district office, are established in suitable locations for the purpose of integrating the state agency program more effectively into community organization and participation.

b. Executive direction and coordination stems from the Director of the Division of Vocational Rehabilitation to the three Bureaus and several consultants.

(1) The Bureau of Rehabilitation Services is responsible for the administration, direction, control and supervision of the State-wide program of direct services to disabled clients. The Bureau Chief is responsible to the Division Director for program planning and coordination, assessment of future needs, and maintenance of high standards of both quantity and quality throughout the state.

(2) The Bureau of Disability Determination administers the program of disability determination under the provisions of the Social Security Act. The Bureau Chief is responsible to the Division Director for carrying out the terms of a formal agreement between the Social Security Administration of the Department of Health, Education, and Welfare, and the Board of Education of the State of Connecticut.

(3) The Bureau of Community and Institutional Services administers the Facility Program for Workshops and Rehabilitation Centers, the Research and Demonstration Projects Program and the Cooperative School Programs. The Bureau Chief is responsible to the Division Director for: (a) The Certification and effective utilization of established rehabilitation centers and workshops, promotion of the growth and development of present facilities, and of new facilities as needed. (b) Consultative services to establish research and demonstration projects and promotion of the growth and development of these projects and of new projects in response to present and future program needs. (c) Administration of the cooperative school programs for services to young handicapped persons and the development and growth of these programs throughout the State through continued cooperation with the Division of Vocational Education, Division of Instructional Services (Department of Education), local school boards and other related agencies.

c. The Consultant for Training and Communications is responsible to the Division Director for the program of public information and program interpretation. This will include:

(1) The publishing of a periodic newsletter to inform the staff and interested persons of activities and new developments in the field of rehabilitation.

(2) The provision of audio-visual materials for staff members to use in their local communities.

(3) Training staff in proper presentation of these materials and provisions of outline speeches.

(4) Development of new opportunities throughout the State for presentation of rehabilitation information.

(5) Preparation and distribution of news releases pertaining to the field of vocational rehabilitation.

d. The Counselor, under the supervision of the District and Local Directors, is responsible for direct services to individual clients. He investigates, evaluates, counsels, plans, and arranges for the provision of needed services, such as physical restoration or training and is responsible for job placement and follow-up to determine the suitability of the placement.

e. The Chief of the Bureau of Community and Institutional Services is responsible for the establishment and utilization of workshops and rehabilitation facilities.

f. Physical Restoration services are provided after approval by the District Medical Consultant, District Psychiatric Consultant, or District Psychological Consultant, as applicable.

g. Consultative Services for special disability groups are secured from appropriate sources as necessary. In many cases, experienced counselors currently serving the particular disability group (i.e., a counselor working full time in a psychiatric hospital) may readily furnish the necessary information.

h. The responsibilities of the Bureau of Disability Determination and Disability Adjudicators in respect to the Division of Vocational Rehabilitation are as follows:

(1) The screening of disability determination cases for vocational rehabilitation potential, and referral of appropriate cases.

(2) The provision of medical, vocational and other data from the case file in conjunction with referrals.

(3) The effective use and development of rehabilitation resources including psychological, medical and vocational areas in coordination with the Division.

(4) The coordination of medical relations and procedures with the Division.

i. Provision of rehabilitation services to beneficiaries of Social Security Trust Funds is underway.

j. The State agency does not contemplate the establishment of any State Agency-managed business enterprises, homebound industries or vending stand programs.

k. The policies covering any State-agency operated rehabilitation facilities or workshops are described in Sections 22 and 23 of the State Plan.

l. District Organization: District Directors are responsible to the Division Director through the Chief of the Bureau of Rehabilitation Services for the operation and administration of a district office and of the local offices established within the area served by the district office. The District Director plans, directs and supervises the rehabilitation program within the district; plans and operates the district office budget and is responsible for maintenance of accurate fiscal records of the transactions within the district office area.

Local Directors are responsible to the District Director for: Advising counselors in respect to planning and scheduling of work, methods of handling cases and availability of services to most client needs; reviewing flow sheets and other caseload control devices; and supervising the development of sound individual rehabilitation plans.

m. Statistical reports are received monthly from the district offices, covering such items as referral sources, number of referrals, new cases accepted, types of disability, status numbers, closures, etc. The Central Office collects and analyzes this information and prepares statistical reports from the federal and state governments, and for use in budgeting and public information activities.

A Statistical Research Project has also been established which is studying the use of computers in tabulating and analyzing this type of information, and is developing new methods of compiling information at the district office level.

Next year will be the final for this $100,000 five (5) year project.
n. Accounting, budget and fiscal activities are described in sections 4.3 and 4.4 of the State Plan.

As important as this has been in the past, the Connecticut Vocational Rehabilitation Agency of the future must be much more effective in providing statewide and community leadership in the identification of the needs of handicapped people and in developing and delivering leadership responsibility, and in evaluating vocational rehabilitation services. The new Vocational Rehabilitation Act has placed on State Vocational Rehabilitation agencies specific leadership responsibilities which include:

1. *Administration and supervision* of an expanded program of direct vocational rehabilitation services to handicapped citizens (underway).
2. *Statewide planning* leading toward the provision by 1975 of comprehensive, high-quality vocational rehabilitation services to all who need them. Although the authority for making these studies is vested in the State, vocational rehabilitation agencies are being entrusted with the responsibility in most states (underway).
3. *Developing a state plan* for an adequate network of rehabilitation facilities and workshops to serve handicapped people (underway).
4. *Working with local communities in developing plans for establishing and staffing workshops and rehabilitation facilities* and acting on applications of local communities for federal funds to support local projects (underway).
5. Providing consultative services to workshops in the development of workshop improvement and technical service projects and recommending approval of such projects to the Secretary of Health, Education, and Welfare (underway).
6.*Providing consultative services to workshops and rehabilitation facilities* that may be used for special training programs to be supported by Federal funds, certification of handicapped individuals as eligible for such training services, and certifying that workshops meet standards set by the Secretary (underway).
7. *Consultation with community organizations in developing research and demonstration projects* and the approval of such projects when they involve direct services to handicapped people (underway).

Harbridge House Study of
Vocational Rehabilitation

To implement plans and formulations by out own staff, the Harbridge House Study of Vocational Rehabilitation includes certain recommendations which have implications for the 1967-1969 budget. They are:

1. The client service capacity of the division should be increased six-fold to provide for the rehabilitation of approximately 6,000 persons a year, a level that approximates the estimated gross annual increment of potentially eligible cases of disability in the state.

2. In view of the administrative and organizational problems that are attendant upon such an expansion, this increase in capacity can be expected to be attained no earlier than 1971.

3. The capacity of rehabilitation facilities in Connecticut should be substantially increased in response to the proposed increase in client service capacity.

4. The additional facilities program should specifically include:

a. Training and rehabilitation facilities and units, to the number of several hundred a year, at existing state institutions and state penal institutions for the mentally retarded and mentally ill.

b. In-patient workshop and training facilities at existing rehabilitation hospitals sufficient to serve several hundred patients a year.

c. The expansion of existing private comprehensive rehabilitation facilities and sheltered workshops by an amount providing for the services of several hundred clients a year.

d. The development of a new major rehabilitation center in Connecticut that would:

(1) Be sponsored and operated by the Division.

(2) Serve clients with a wide range of disabilities.

(3) Provide a comprehensive program of services emphasizing vocational training rather than medical care.

(4) Offer both in-patient and out-patient care.

(5) Be located near a major urban center.

(6) Have the capacity to serve several hundred seriously disabled clients a year.

e. The provision of residential half-way houses for those persons who need a partially supportive environment in making the transition from institutional life to competitive employment and for those who require such a supportive environment indefinitely. The number of places afforded should be several hundred.

5. In response to the proposed increase in client service capacity, the professional staff of the Division should be increased six-fold to a total of approximately *120 field staff by 1971.*

6. An increase in total funding that is more than proportionate to the proposed increase in client service capacity should be sought. The minimum annual level of funding necessary to support a client service capacity of 6,000 cases per year in 1971 is $5 million. An annual level of funding of $7.2 million is desirable and probably will be necessary.

7. The increase in funding should be found by:

a. An increase in the annual level of state appropriations to at least $1.5 million and preferably $1.8 million.

b. A corresponding increase in Federal matching funds to at least $4.5 million annually, and preferably to $5.4 million.

c. The employment of categorical Federal grants for:

(1) Assistance in construction and equipment of rehabilitation facilities.

(2) In-service training of professional staff.

(3) Long-term program planning.

(4) Special research and demonstration projects.

d. The use of third-party financing to capture further Federal funds for cooperative programs.

8. The present practice of appropriating State funds for a particular rehabilitation purpose should be abandoned.

Citizen's Advisory Committee

To assist in guiding the extension and improvement of the rehabilitation program, a Citizen's Advisory Committee was established by the State Board of Education at its meeting of December 1, 1965.

Bureau of Rehabilitation Services

The planned total anticipated expenditure program for the Bureau of Rehabilitation Services during fiscal 1966 amounted to approximately $2,000,000, of which the federal portion was $1,250,000, and state matching funds were $750,000. This represents an increase of approximately 2 1/2 times the actual expenditures made for rehabilitation program purposes in fiscal 1965. In 1965, expenditures of both federal and state funds totaled $847,048.

As of June 1, 1966 the size of the staff of the Bureau of Rehabilitation Services was increased by twenty professional and thirteen clerical workers. Based upon statistical evidence covering the six-month period, July 1, 1965 - December 31, 1965, the Bureau of Rehabilitation Services' caseload for the entire fiscal year is estimated below:

Referrals received	3,650
Referrals Processed	2,500
Referrals awaiting processing	1,150
Total inactive load	5,000
Closed rehabilitated	1,300
Closed other reasons	200
Total active cases remaining at end of year	3,000

Bureau of Disability Determination

During the period July 1, 1965 through April 30, 1966, the Bureau completed the processing of 5364 cases. The number of new cases received during this period was 5384. There were 344 pending cases at the beginning of the fiscal year. The remainder of the fiscal year will bring in approximately 1100 cases. Therefore, the total caseload for the year is estimated to be 6484. By the end of the fiscal year 6134 cases will have been adjudicated. The expenditures for the fiscal year will approximate $313,000.

What could not be clearly perceived in 1963, was the continuing upswing in nationwide concern relative to Federal and State action on social and economic problems of individuals and families who were out of the mainstream of our society. The forward thrust, led by the "Negro Revolt" jarred us out of our state of inertia and propelled us into concerned action on behalf of the deprived.

In order to make our Public Law 89-333 program function properly for the deprived, we must not forget that for the first time "physical or mental disability" is defined to include "behavior disorders characterized by deviant social behavior or impaired ability to carry out normal relationships with family and community which may result from *vocational, educational, cultural, social, environmental*, or other factors." The above factors are also to apply in determining whether the handicapped individual has a substantial handicap for gainful employment. Gainful employment includes farm or family work without cash payment, sheltered employment, and home employment.

The implication of the above definition for the State VR agencies is profound in nation. In many respects the average client will be more severely disabled and many more cases with behavioral, educational, social, and cultural deprivation problems will make up our caseloads. Many more, definitive services of a vocational rehabilitation mold, operationally, will have to be evaluated for personal and social adjustment and basic educational services. It is now possible for these services to precede the determination as to whether the individual can be rehabilitated at all. The chronic alcoholic, the public offender, the narcotic addict, the unwed mother, the functional illiterate, the mentally restored, the unskilled welfare recipient, and the retarded, to name a few, may be eligible without relating their problems to medically determined physical or mental disability or to a prescribed intelligence measurement or IQ.

Now that we are free of the legal straitjacket that boxed us in for over forty years, we need help from you, the consumers of our services, to aid us as we group our forces for the final victory over deprivation in this era of "The Great Society."

ॐ

CHAPTER FOURTEEN

REHABILITATION'S RESPONSIBILITY
TO THE DISADVANTAGED

James S. Peters, II, Ph.D.
Director, Division of Vocational Rehabilitation
Connecticut State Department of Education

One of the most challenging and far-reaching changes in social, welfare, health and education legislation in recent years came about through the vocational Rehabilitation Act Amendments (P.L. 89-333) passed by the Congress during its 1965 session. These amendments were the instrumentation for greatly strengthening the program of vocational rehabilitation of the physically and mentally handicapped and also making the socio-cultural disadvantaged eligible for the vocational rehabilitation services. Now with Section 15 of the Vocational Rehabilitation Act of 1968 we have a tremendous opportunity to help remove the scars of segregation and discrimination from the "soul" and backs of America's Blacks and other deprived minorities, as well as the socio-culturally handicapped.

The new Grants-in-Aid programs to workshops, rehabilitation facilities, as well as other public and private non-profit Health, Education, and Welfare agencies are enabling our program to capture more federal funds and plan better programs in our efforts to help the state of Connecticut to eradicate those twin enemies of progress—poverty and dependency.

A talk given for the Lion's Club of Hartford, Thursday, June 1, 1967, Shoreham Motor Hotel, Hartford, Connecticut.
Given before meeting of State Directors, Vocational Rehabilitation and Region I of Vocational Rehabilitation personnel, Sheraton Biltmore Hotel, New England Regional Conference National Rehabilitation Association, Providence, Rhode Island, June 13, 1967.
Given at the training institute conducted by the Massachusetts and Connecticut Chapters of the National Association of Sheltered Workshops and Homebound Programs, Heritage House Motor Hotel, Hyannis, Massachusetts, April 22, 1969.

When Governor John Dempsey signed into law House Bill 3139, "An Act Establishing a Division of Vocational Rehabilitation with the State Department of Education," on Wednesday, June 2, 1965, along with Congress he sealed the end of legislative discrimination against groups just as handicapped as "the lame, the halt, and the blind," i.e., the deprived American Negro and other racial, ethnic, and sociological minorities. The later characterized as jail inmates, juvenile delinquents, drug addicts, homosexuals, unwed mothers, school dropouts, etc. Through a new Bill (H. 13-649), in our 1965 legislation, we will have a mandate to go much farther in our quest to make tax producers out of tax recipients; to make solid citizens of the ne'er-do-well, to make skilled and semi-skilled workers of the classical "hewers-of-wood and drawers-of-water." The major limitations of such a far reaching idealized version of our role in State and Federal financing or funding. There are many minor limitations of such a far reaching idealized version of our role in State and Federal financing or funding. There are many minor limitations that "we could overcome" if we could come to grips with the former. This bill, "An Act Concerning Vocational Rehabilitation," has received a favorable hearing before a joint Senate and House Committee and is now scheduled to be acted upon by the General Assembly. In the event of its passage, I am certain that the Governor will sign it for he has, more than any other Chief Executive of the State of Connecticut, as well as his administrative aides, demonstrated his interest in all of Connecticut's citizens and, in particular, those disadvantaged by birth defects, environments, deprivation, disease, race, religion, inadequate education and, you name it, our Governor is interested. He is, and have no doubts about it, one of the greatest humanitarians in contemporary public life.

It might interest those of you present if I read the major provisions of our Act. It begins with the Statement of Purpose: (see appendix)

For the fiscal years 1970 and 1971 the Governor has recommended for approval all of the money we requested, $1,204,178 (this included fringe benefits) making a total of $2,258,386 for the bi-annum. If the General Assembly approves these amounts, we stand in a good position to capture all available federal funds. This will enable us to increase greatly our Workshop and Facilities Program which is under the supervision of Clifford Beebe, our Consultant and Specialist, who is doing a great job in this area. He, and his co-workers, are aware of the need to meet the challenge of the Vocational Rehabilitation of the disadvantaged.

The Division of Vocational Rehabilitation will rehabilitate to gainful employment over 2,000 disabled men and women this year, although we work with many more. Only four years ago, we were rehabilitating less than 1,000 disabled persons per year. Lest we rest on our recent progress and become too self-satisfied, according to a recently completed administrative study of vocational rehabilitation in Connecticut by the Harbridge House, Inc. Consulting Firm (March, 1966), there is need for rehabilitating 6,000 disabled persons per year by fiscal year 1971 if we are to keep pace with growth and development of program needs in the state. We are striving to obtain this goal.

It is our intention to forge ahead, and especially into the area where the action is, the area of what Michael Harrington so aptly calls, "The Other America," the world of the socio-cultural disadvantaged where we are witnessing many behavioral problems; especially in the urban communities. This is a new challenge for vocational rehabilitation. According to Harrington:

> In the past, when poverty was general in the unskilled and semi-skilled work force, the poor were all mixed together. The bright and those who were going to stay behind, all of them lived on the same street. When the middle third rose, this community was destroyed and the entire invisible land of the other America became a ghetto, a modern poor farm of rejects of society and of the economy...

Galbraith was one of the first writers to begin to describe the newness of contemporary poverty, and that is to his credit. Yet, because even he underestimated the problem, it is important to put his definition into perspective.

For Galbraith, there are two major components of the new poverty: case poverty and insular poverty. Case poverty is the plight of those who suffer from some physical disability or mental disability that is personal and individual and excluded them from the general advance.

Insular poverty exists in areas like the Appalachians or the West Virginia coal fields, where an entire section of the country becomes economically obsolete.

Keeping in mind the components of the new poverty, case poverty and insular poverty, as described by Dr. Galbraith, we are now ready to advance a new component which we shall tentatively call *sensori-perceptual poverty*.

By sensori-perceptual poverty, we mean poverty which results from, or is caused by sensory and perceptual deprivation through poor housing, segregated and inferior education, job discrimination, minimum access to cultural stimulation and overriding feelings of alienation, rejection and isolation from the mainstream of society. Such sociological and psychological patterns blunt sensory stimuli and color perceptual cues, thereby creating within the individual pathological symptoms more indicative of what Karen Horney called, "the neurotic personality of our time," or what the military psychologists classified as undifferentiated neurosis or psychosis. This is a behavioral manifestation. To quote Harrington:

> Physical and mental disabilities are, to be sure, an important part of poverty in America. The poor are sick in body and in spirit. But this is not an isolated fact about them, an individual 'case,' a stroke of bad luck. Disease, alcoholism, low IQ's, these express a whole way of life. They are, in the main, the effects of an environment, not the biographies of the unlucky individuals. Because of this, the new poverty is something that cannot be dealt with by first aid. If there is to be lasting assault on the shame of the other America, it must seek to root out of this society an entire environment and not just the relief of individuals.

Through our new Vocational Rehabilitation Cooperative School Programs, Correction Programs, Programs for the Mentally Restored and the Retardates, etc., we are endeavoring to bring more relief to the handicapped individual; we are bringing him hope. Hope of a better tomorrow and the mechanisms for achieving. The young Negro, the Puerto Rican, the retardate especially needs this hope, for they live in a perpetual ghetto of collective human indignities in the form of mass hate, alienation and rejection. Those individuals who are able to rise above this cauldron of reactions are the exceptional ones. But many are to be scarred psychologically, and need specialized services help through rehabilitation and other agencies. As Samuel D. Proctor, Special Assistant to the Director of the Peace Corps, writes in "The Young Negro in America, 1960-1980."

> Under the most favorable conditions, the young Negro will find it a real task to overcome his educational deficit, change the poverty pattern and outline the American stereotype of the Negro. If he plays for keeps, he will succeed; and in 1980, he will look back and see that he has come a long way. Hopefully, those who are

now managers and leaders may share in this appraisal and help forge the framework for a true democracy in America.

The Connecticut Vocational Rehabilitation Agency is providing state-wide and community leadership in the identification of the needs of disadvantaged people and is developing guidelines and cooperative programs with the Welfare Department, Department of Community Affairs, Department of Personnel, Model Cities Programs and Community Action based programs of vocational rehabilitation services. The new Vocational Rehabilitation Acts, State and Federal, have placed on State Vocational Rehabilitation agencies specific leadership responsibilities which includes.

1. *Administration and Supervision* of an extended program of direct Vocational Rehabilitation Services to handicapped citizens (underway).
2. *State-wide planning* leading toward the provision by 1975 of comprehensive, and high quality vocational rehabilitation services to all who need them. Although the authority for making these studies is vested in the State, through the Governor, our agency is being entrusted with the responsibility.
3. *Developing a state plan* for an adequate network of rehabilitation facilities and workshops to serve handicapped people.
4. *Working with local communities in developing plans for establishing and staffing workshops and rehabilitation facilities* and acting on applications of local communities for federal funds to support local projects.
5. *Providing consultative services to workshops* in the development of workshop improvement and technical service projects and recommending approval of such projects to the Secretary of Health, Education, and Welfare. (Second year completed.)
6. *Providing consultative services to workshops and rehabilitation facilities* that may be used for special training programs to be supported by federal funds, certification of handicapped individuals as eligible for such training services, and certifying that workshops meet standards set by the Secretary.
7. *Consultation with community organizations in developing research and demonstration projects* and the approval of such projects when they involve direct services to handicapped people.

If the Connecticut Vocational Rehabilitation Agency is to perform this leadership role effectively, its personnel and organization must reflect the scope of its responsibilities.

Not only must its Director be a leader of stature, vision and administrative skill and courage, he must also have the administrative and technical assistance that is required to enable an agency to work effectively with rehabilitation centers, workshops, schools, hospitals, colleges, and universities in providing rehabilitation services.

To implement plans and formulations by our own staff, the Harbridge House study of Vocational Rehabilitation included certain recommendations which had implications for 1967-1969 budget. They are:

1. The client service capacity of the Division should be increased six-fold to provide for the rehabilitation of approximately 6,000 persons a year, a level that approximates the estimated gross annual increment of potentially eligible cases of disability in the state.

2. In view of the administrative and organizational problems that are attendant upon such an expansion, this increase in capacity can be expected to be attained no earlier than 1971.

3. The capacity of rehabilitation facilities in Connecticut should be substantially increased to respond to the proposed increase in client service capacity.

4. The additional facilities program should specifically include:

a. Training and rehabilitation facilities and units, to the number of several hundred a year, at existing state institutions and state penal institutions for the mentally retarded and mentally ill.

b. In-patient workshop and training facilities at existing rehabilitation hospitals sufficient to serve several hundred clients a year.

c. The expansion of existing private comprehensive rehabilitation facilities and sheltered workshops by an amount providing for the service of several hundred clients a year.

d. The development of new major rehabilitation center in Connecticut that would:

(1) Be sponsored and operated by the Division.

(2) Serve clients with a wide range of disabilities.

(3) Provide a comprehensive program of services emphasizing vocational training rather than medical care.

(4) Offer both in-patient and out-patient care.

(5) Be located near a major urban center.

(6) Have the capacity to serve several hundred seriously disabled clients a year.

e. The provision of residential half-way houses for these persons who need a partially supportive environment in making the transition from institutional life to competitive employment and for those who require such a supportive environment indefinitely. The number of places afforded should be several hundred.

5. In response to the proposed increase in client service capacity, the professional staff of the Division should be increased six-fold to a total of approximately 120 field staff by 1971.

6. An increase in total funding that is more than proportionate to the proposed increase in client service capacity should be sought. The minimum annual level of funding necessary to support a client service capacity of 6,000 cases per year in 1971 is $6 million. An annual level of funding of 7.2 million dollars is desirable and probably will be necessary.

7. The increase in funding should be found by:

a. An increase in the annual level of State appropriations to at least $1.5 million and preferably 1.8 million dollars.

b. A corresponding increase in Federal matching funds to at last 4.5 million dollars annually, and preferably to 5.4 million dollars.

c. The employment of categorical Federal grants for:

(1)Assistance in construction and equipment of rehabilitation facilities.

(2)In-service training of professional staff.

(3)Long-term program planning.

(4)Special research and demonstration projects.

d. The use of third-party financing to capture further Federal funds for cooperative programs.

8. The present practice of appropriating State funds of a particular rehabilitation purpose should be abandoned.

To assist in guiding the extension and improvement of the rehabilitation program, a Citizens Advisory Committee was established by the State Board of Education in December, 1965. The Committee met twice a year; once in the fall and again in the spring. The Executive Committee met with the Division Director more frequently. This Committee's work was taken over by the State Planning Council for Vocational Rehabilitation Services during the phase of State-wide Planning. This Council was chaired by Attorney Joseph W. Kess of West Hartford whose work is now complete, and the findings and recommendations are now before the State's Planning Council which was formed by the Governor.

It has been said by experts in rehabilitation that "a civilization may be measured in some degree by the treatment accorded the disabled members of its society." Among certain past civilizations, such practices as putting the disabled to death or locking them away were followed. Even in this country, the disabled have not always been accorded the best treatment. However, in our times, their talents are being recognized, and they are being brought "out of the closets" and "off the shelves" and through the doorways to opportunity which have been opened by a more enlightened and informed citizenry.

THE STATE OF VOCATIONAL REHABILITATION IN CONNECTICUT

James S. Peters, II, Ph.D.
Director, Division of Vocational Rehabilitation
Connecticut State Department of Education

One of the most challenging and far-reaching changes in social, welfare, health and education legislation in recent years came about through the Vocational Rehabilitation Act Amendments (PL 89-333) passed by the Congress during its 1965 session. These amendments were the instrumentation for greatly strengthening the program of vocational rehabilitation of the physically and mentally handicapped and also making the socio-cultural disadvantage eligible for the various vocational rehabilitation services.

The new Grants-In-Aid Program to workshops, rehabilitation facilities, as well as other public and private non-profit Health, Education and Welfare Agencies is enabling our program to capture more federal funds and plan better programs in our efforts to help the State of Connecticut to eradicate those twin enemies of progress-poverty and dependency.

When Governor John Dempsey signed into law House Bill 3139, "An Act Establishing a Division of Vocational Rehabilitation within the State Department of Education," on Wednesday, June 2, 1956, along with Congress, he sealed the end of legislative discrimination against groups

A talk given to Employ the Handicapped Committee of Greater Bridgeport, October 9, 1967.
Given at Conference for Federal Coordination of Handicapped, Hartford, Connecticut, October 19, 1967.
Given at the 10th Annual Meeting of the Waterbury Area Rehabilitation Center, Waterbury, Connecticut, December 7, 1967.

just as handicapped as "the lame," the halt, and the blind," i.e., the deprived American Negro and other racial, ethnic and sociological minorities. The latter are characterized as jail inmates, juvenile delinquents, drug addicts, homosexuals, unwed mothers, school dropouts, etc. No type of handicapped person is left out of this new legislation. We have the mandate to go forward in our quest to make tax producers out of tax recipients; to make solid citizens of the ne'er-do-well; to make skilled and semi-skilled workers of the classical "hewers-of-wood and drawers-of-water." The major limitation of such a far-reaching idealized version of our role is state financing or funding. There are many minor limitations that "we could overcome" if we could come to grips with the former.

With the greatly increased budget for vocational rehabilitation services during the present biennium, our program has broadened and improved considerably. For example, for this fiscal year, 1967, the state's appropriation is $904,000. The federal appropriation, which is now 75% of our budget, will come to approximately $2,712,000, making a total of $3,616,000 available. For the next biennium, we requested from the legislature, $1,901,738 to match an allotment from the Vocational Rehabilitation Administration, Department of Health, Education and Welfare, of $5,700,620, making a total state and federal allocation for Vocational Rehabilitation Services of $7,602,358 (1968-1969). However, the legislature only appropriated $800,000 for fiscal 1968, and $900,000 for fiscal 1969, making a total of $1,700,000 to match funds from the federal government. For fiscal 1968 we will have $15,000 from the Social Security Trust Fund to match our $800,000. This gives us a total of $815,000. ($808,822 will be Section 2 money for matching $2,426,466 federal grant). Approximately $3,100,000 is available to Connecticut. Our share is $2,700,000, and the agency for the blind, $300,000. We will be unable to match nearly $300,000 unless the third-party financing method is made operative.

The Division of Vocational Rehabilitation will rehabilitate to gainful employment some 1552 disabled men and women this year, although we work with many more. Only two years ago, we were rehabilitating less than 1,000 disabled persons per year. Lest we rest on our recent progress and become too self-satisfied, according to a recently completed administrative study of vocational rehabilitation in Connecticut by the Harbridge House, Inc., Consulting Firm (March, 1966), there is a need for rehabilitating 6,000 disabled persons per year by fiscal year 1971 if we are to keep pace with growth and development of program needs in the state. According to a report from Mr. A. Ryrie Koch, Regional Assistant Commissioner of Vocational Rehabilitation, Region I Office, Department of Health,

Education and Welfare, Boston, Massachusetts, Connecticut is leading the region in percent of rehabilitation over last year. It is our intention to forge ahead, and especially into the area where the action is, the area of what Michael Harrington so aptly calls, "The Other America," the world of the socio-cultural disadvantaged where we are witnessing many behavioral problems, especially in the urban communities. This is a new challenge for vocational rehabilitation. According to Harrington:

> In the past, when poverty was general in the unskilled and semi-skilled work force, the poor were all mixed together. The bright and those who were going to stay behind, all of them lived on the same street. When the middle third rose, this community was destroyed and the entire invisible land of the other America became a ghetto, a modern poor farm of the rejects of society and of the economy...

Galbraith was one of the first writers to begin to describe the newness of contemporary poverty, and that is to his credit. Yet because even he underestimates the problem it is important to put his definition into perspective.

For Galbraith, there are two main components of the new poverty: case poverty and insular poverty. Case poverty is the plight of those who suffer from some physical or mental disability that is personal and individual and excludes them from the general advance. Insular poverty exists in areas like the Appalachians or the West Virginia coal fields, where an entire section of the country becomes economically obsolete.

Keeping in mind the components of the new poverty, case poverty and insular poverty, as described by Dr. Galbraith, we are now ready to advance a new component which we shall tentatively call *sensori-perceptual poverty.*

By *sensori-perceptual poverty,* we mean poverty which results from, or is caused by, sensory and perceptual deprivation through poor housing, segregated and inferior education, job discrimination, minimum access to cultural stimulation and overriding feelings of alienation, rejection and isolation from the mainstream of society. Such sociological and psychological patterns blunt sensory stimuli and color perceptual; cues, thereby creating within the individual pathological symptoms more indicative of what Karen Horney called, "the neurotic personality of our time," or what the military psychologists classified as, undifferentiated neurosis or psychosis. This is a behavioral manifestation. To again quote Harrington:

Under the most favorable conditions, the young Negro will find it a real task to overcome his educational deficit, change the poverty pattern and outlive the American stereotype of the Negro. If he plays for keeps, he will succeed; and in 1980, he will look back and see that he has come a long way. Hopefully, those who are now managers and leaders may share in this appraisal and help forge the framework for a true democracy in America.

The Connecticut Vocational Rehabilitation agency is providing statewide and community leadership in the identification of the needs of handicapped people and in developing and evaluating vocational rehabilitation services. The new Vocational Rehabilitation Act has placed on State Vocational Rehabilitation agencies specific leadership responsibilities which include:

1.*Administration and supervision* of an extended program of direct vocational rehabilitation services to handicapped citizens (underway)

2.*Statewide planning* leading toward the provision by 1975 of comprehensive, high quality vocational rehabilitation services to all who need them.

Although the authority for making these studies is vested in the state, through the Governor, our agency is being entrusted with the responsibility. Connecticut is the only state in the region so designated. (1st year completed.)

3. *Developing a state plan. for* an adequate network of rehabilitation facilities and workshops to serve handicapped people (1st year completed)- Plan approved by VRA subject to a few minor modifications.

4. *Working with local communities in developing plans for establishing and staffing workshops and rehabilitation facilities* and acting on applications of local communities for federal funds to support loan projects (1st year completed).

5. *Providing consultative services to workshops* in the development of workshop improvement and technical service projects and recommending approval of such projects to the Secretary of Health, Education and Welfare (1st year completed).

6. *Providing consultative services to workshops and rehabilitation facilities* that may be used for special training programs to be

supported by federal funds, certifications of handicapped individuals as eligible for such training services, and certifying that workshops meet standards set by the Secretary (1st year completed).

7. *Consultation with community organizations in developing research and demonstration projects* and the approval of such projects when the involve direct services to handicapped people (1st year completed).

If the Connecticut Vocational Rehabilitation Agency is to perform this leadership role effectively, its personnel and organization must reflect the scope of its responsibilities.

Not only must its director be a leader of stature, vision and administrative skill and courage, he must also have the administrative and technical assistance that is required to enable an agency to work effectively with rehabilitation centers, workshops, schools, hospitals, colleges and universities in providing rehabilitation services.

To implement plans and formulations by our own staff, the Harbridge House study of Vocational Rehabilitation includes certain recommendations which have implications for the 1967-1969 budget. They are:

1.The client service capacity of the Division should be increased six-fold to provide for the rehabilitation of approximately 6,000 persons a year, a level that approximates the estimated gross annual increment of potentially eligible cases of disability in the state.

2.In view of the administrative and organizational problems that are attendant upon such an expansion, this increase in capacity can be expected to be attained no earlier than 1971.

3. The capacity of rehabilitation facilities in Connecticut should be substantially increased to respond to the proposed increase in client service capacity.

4. The additional facilities program should specifically include:

a. Training and rehabilitation facilities and units, to the number of several hundred a year, at existing state institutions and state penal institutions for the mentally retarded and mentally ill.

b. In-patient workshop and training facilities at existing rehabilitation hospitals sufficient to serve several hundred clients a year.

c. The expansion of existing private comprehensive rehabilitation facilities and sheltered workshops by an amount providing for the service of several hundred clients a year.

d. The development of a new major rehabilitation center in Connecticut that would:

> (1) Be sponsored and operated by the Division.
> (2)Serve clients with a wide range of disabilities.
> (3) Provide a comprehensive program of services emphasizing vocational training rather than medical care.
> (4) Offer both in-patient and out-patient care.
> (5) Be located near a major urban center.
> (6) Have the capacity to serve several hundred seriously disabled clients a year.

e.The provision of residential half-way houses for these persons who need a partially supportive environment in making the transition from institutional life to competitive employment and for those who require such a supportive environment indefinitely. The number of places afforded should be several hundred.

5. In response to the proposed increase in client service capacity, the professional staff of the Division should be increased six-fold to a total of approximately *120 field staff by 1971.*

6. An increase in total funding that is more than proportionate to the proposed increase in client service capacity should be sought. The minimum annual level of funding necessary to support a client service capacity of 6,000 cases per year in 1971 is $6 million. An annual level of funding of 7.2 million dollars is desirable and probably will be necessary.

7. The increase in funding should be found by:

> a. An increase in the annual level of state appropriations to at least $1.5 million and preferably 1.8 million dollars.
> b. A corresponding increase in Federal matching funds to at least 4.5 million dollars annually, and preferably to 5.4 million dollars.
> c. The employment of categorical Federal grants for:
>> (1)Assistance in construction and equipment of reha-bilitation facilities.
>> (2)In-service training of professional staff.
>> (3)Long-term, program planning.
>> (4)Special research and demonstration projects.

d. The use of third-party financing to capture further Federal funds for cooperative programs.

8. The present practice of appropriating State funds for a particular rehabilitation purpose should be abandoned. To assist in guiding the extension and improvement of the rehabilitation program, a Citizens' Advisory Committee was established by the State Board of Education in December, 1965. The Committee meets twice a year; once in the fall and again in the spring. Its executive committee meets with the Division Director more frequently.

The Committee consists of: John Allen, M.D., Hartford; Mr. Herbert A. Anderson, New Haven; Mrs. David N. Bates, Woodstock; Mr. William M. Cowell, Stamford; Dr. H. Philip Dinan, Bridgeport, Mrs. Glenn Farmer, Old Saybrook; Mr. Cyrus D. Flanders, Wethersfield, Mr. E. Clayton Gengras, West Hartford; Mr. Richard D. Keller, Bloomfield; Dr. Ruby Jo Reeves Kennedy, Waterford; Mr. Carmine R. Lavieri, Winsted; Sidney Licht, M.D., New Haven, Mr. H. Kenneth McCollam, Hartford; Dr. John P. McIntosh, Kensington, Miss Gertrude Norcross, Hartford, Rev. Joseph Pouliot, Bridgeport; Mr. Joseph Ress, Hartford, Chairman; Mr. Carmen Romano, New Haven, and Mr. William S. Simpson, Stratford. The Committee has been very active during the year. Its Chairman, Mr. Ress, has been a leader in our effort to maintain our present position within the Department of education, as well as helpful in other matters.

It has been said by experts in rehabilitation that "a civilization may be measured in some degree by the treatment accorded the disabled members of its society." Among certain past civilizations, such practices as putting the disabled to death or "locking them away" were followed. Even in this country, the disabled have not always been accorded the best treatment. However, in our times, their talents are being recognized, and they are being brought "out of the closets" and "off the shelves" and through the doorways to opportunity which have been opened by a more enlightened and informed citizenry.

CHAPTER SIXTEEN

FREEDOM AND WORK

James S. Peters, II, Ph.D.
Associate Commissioner
Division of Vocational Rehabilitation
Connecticut State Department of Education

To paraphrase an old saying "Work may not make us rich but it will make us free," I address you young men and women this evening because you epitomize this ancient thought. You have, by any stretch of the imagination, weathered the storm of determination and grind in order to take your place among others in the community who are free to pursue the American dream of independence. I congratulate you in this hour of your greatest triumph.

The State of Connecticut, the parents and friends of retardates, the Federal government, all come in for a special thanks for having, through programming and funding at the New Haven Regional Center; produced and packaged a product of human flesh and blood in the person of our honorees, that is salable on the employment market in open competition with other workers. This, to me, represents a far greater achievement than sending a man to the moon; a rocket around the world; a submarine to the bottom of the sea, and tens of thousands to protect our freedom in South East Asia. The greatest need for Americans of today is to create, through programs such as we have at the regional center, opportunities for all Americans to learn the art and skill of work so that they might become useful citizens and take their place among others in a free and open society. We are sick and tired of the pretensions of our scientific and technological endeavors at the expense of human and humane efforts. If the government could give the center one-tenth of the cost of building a rocket, manned or unmanned, who gives a damn, it could produce ten times the number of graduates.

A talk given at banquet honoring community-employed young adults of Regional Center, New Haven, Connecticut, Holiday Inn, May 15, 1970.

However, it is not my purpose this evening to lament our lack of funds but to praise our progress. Again, to quote an old saying, "We have come a long way." Yes, we have come a long way since the initial efforts to bring the retardates into the community and out of the walls of homes and institutions. Many of these earlier efforts were begun right here in New Haven through the cooperation of the New Haven School system, Connecticut Association for Retarded Children, the Division of Vocational Rehabilitation and other agencies and businesses. Let me cite results of one such earlier program.

In an attempt to bridge the gap between school and work, several state and private agencies, including the Bureau of Vocational Rehabilitation, were invited to work out a program of work-school for the retardates.

Thirty-four special education students with IQ's of 50 to 79 who were to graduate the following June made up the first group to be included in a three-year program. Each of the 34 was asked by the rehabilitation counselor in September to list, in order of preference, three types of occupations he would like to go into after graduation. These simple lists became the guide for each individual's future.

An initial interview was followed by individual weekly conferences. Records of academic achievement, extracurricular activities, and psychological evaluations were noted. Guidance directors, guidance counselors, classroom instructors, nurses, placement officers and members of the individual's immediate family were consulted in formulating a vocational plan for each student.

Plans were broken down simply as: (1) training, mainly vocational (i.e., nurse's aide and hairdressing); (2) training, mainly on the job (i.e., welding and auto body repair); (3) military service; (4) placement only; (5) no plans. Since this proved to be a workable system, it was used for each succeeding class. The vocational results of each class group and each follow-up presented some enlightening information.

First and foremost was the variety of job classifications defined in the *Dictionary of Occupational Titles* for which the clients were trained. As described in the November, 1964, newsletter of the President's Committee on Employment of the Handicapped:

"From drummer to barber, with 49 kinds of jobs in between—that's the employment record of 91 retarded young people who graduated from a special work-school program in New Haven, Connecticut, over the past three years. More than half the jobs demanded some skills. Further, of the 91, only eight had switched jobs. Of the eight, three changed only once while five changed more than once. Of the five, three were short-order cooks who had to switch jobs with the season, city in winter, resorts in summer. The key to successful placements was that the retardates were considered man-to-man as human beings with human dignity, and not as look-alike, act alike "cases," says James S. Peters and Henry J. Rohde of Connecticut's Division of Vocational Rehabilitation, in a paper presented at the American Personnel and Guidance Association Convention. For example, each retardate was placed in a small business, so he wouldn't "get lost in the crowd" of a big enterprise. Each was treated as an individual, in need of a little help in order to become a useful citizen, earning his own way, raising his own family, paying his own taxes. Each was asked for the kind of work he wanted to do after completing his training—and whenever possible his wishes were respected. One young man, for example, said he wanted to be a drummer. This was respected as his sincere choice and not as a "pie-in-the-sky" dream. He was given music lessons. Today, he heads a jazz combo booked solidly for weeks in advance... Still another example, one fine athlete with a performance level above 100 but a verbal level below 70 has been snapped up by a semi-pro football team; he's an outstanding success..."

Now as we move forward into a "Brave New World" for all disadvantaged and handicapped people, we stand by our creed that work is a right that all citizens who are qualified, should have. When this right is violated we are guilty of denying opportunity of independence to so many of our deserving people. We must continue to seek this right to work in the spirit of the poet James Russell Lowell:

Once to Every Man and Nation

Once to every man and nation
Comes the moment to decide
In the strife of Truth with Falsehood
For the good or evil side

By the light of burning martyrs,
Jesus' bleeding feet I track,
Toiling up new Calvaries ever
With the cross that turns not back.

Though the cause of evil prosper,
Yet 'tis truth alone is strong
Truth forever on the scaffold
Wrong forever on the throne.

Yet the scaffold sways the future,
And behind the dim unknown,
Standeth God within the shadow
Keeping watch above his own.

❦

CHAPTER SEVENTEEN

A NEW PERSPECTIVE IN
REHABILITATION

James S. Peters, II, Ph.D.
Associate Commissioner
Bureau of Vocational Rehabilitation
Connecticut State Department of Education

To the clergy, your Honor the Mayor, Gaylord Farm Association, Dr. Hines and staff, guests and visiting friends, I bring you greetings from the State Department of Education, Division of Vocational Rehabilitation, and Social and Rehabilitation Services, Department of Health and Welfare of our Federal Government. Those of us responsible for vocational rehabilitation services to disabled and handicapped people in the State of Connecticut are pleased to have been afforded the opportunity to be a part of this "New Perspective in Rehabilitation."

On June 1st we will commence the celebration of the fiftieth anniversary of the signing of the Vocational Rehabilitation Act in 1920, thereby making possible federal and state financial support for citizens throughout the country who could not work because of disease or injury. This support allowed for the establishment of programs and services which would serve as a vehicle to render each patient fit to return, or go, to work. Over the years the program has grown and been refined. From its inception, the medical rehabilitation aspect has played a primary role. A guideline for vocational rehabilitation is that the patient must be found medically feasible by a certified physician before he can be accepted for vocational rehabilitation services.

For years we have had an excellent program arrangement for vocational rehabilitation services here at Gaylord. Not only have we afforded

Remarks given at dedication of the Medical Rehabilitation Wing, Elizabeth Russell Hooker, The Gaylord Hospital, Wallingford, Conn., May 23, 1970.

counseling, training, medical and other traditional opportunities for individual patients, but we have participated in conferences, workshops, seminars, etc. and have been a part of the team which designed earlier research and demonstration projects and the packaging of application for grants from Social and Rehabilitation Services, Department of Health, Education and Welfare, to aid in the construction of the vocational workshop and this wonderful new facility.

I am certain that as we move into the second half century of vocational rehabilitation, Gaylord will afford our team of specialists ever-increasing opportunities to aid in the "total rehabilitation" of disabled citizens of the State of Connecticut. Here we have all of the modalities to make this dream possible. We are only limited by adherence to old and outmoded traditions, so let us gear our sights to this new perspective and be on our way to ever-rewarding opportunities in rehabilitation.

CHAPTER EIGHTEEN

VOCATIONAL REHABILITATION AND THE CULTURALLY DEPRIVED MENTALLY RETARDATE

James S. Peters, II, Ph.D.
Associate Commissioner
Division of Vocational Rehabilitation
Connecticut State Department of Education

The State-Federal Vocational Rehabilitation Program for a period of 40 or more years was not known by, and had little relevancy to, minority groups, and in particular American Blacks. Its program was white, middle-class oriented in style and in substance. Prior to the "Black Revolt" and Civil Rights movement of the sixties and the Johnson administration's "War on Poverty," few blacks were employed in the various local, state and federal offices of Vocational Rehabilitation and, worse still, only a small percentage of state agencies case loads were clients who were Black or culturally deprived. Even today, because such a large portion of Blacks fall into the lower socio-economic class (approximately 50%) there are some questions as to the relevancy of vocational rehabilitation services to Black and other minority groups as the program is now structured and/or constituted.

It is important to note that traditional rehabilitation services are being challenged as to their effectiveness in aiding the culturally disadvantaged (Kunce and Cope, 1969). The characteristics of this client-group force a reconsideration of some of the basic assumptions and modes of operation in rehabilitation. Some suggestions concerning rehabilitation counseling with such disadvantaged clients can be made:

A talk given at the National Urban League Project "Star" Training program, April 1, 1971, Tampa, Florida

(1) Traditional one-to one counseling relying heavily upon the relationship, per se, is not sufficient. Lewis Mumford, one of the great non-academic minds of our time, has written widely on such diverse subjects as civilization, culture, cities, conditions of man, etc. Although he never received a college degree, he is a member of The American Philosophical Society and The National Institute of Arts and Letters, and a Fellow of The American Academy of Arts and Science. Mr. Mumford has this to say in his recently published opus "The Pentagon of Power":

> There is always a disparity between ideal professions and actual achievements, at very least, a gap in time. This is part of the natural history of human institutions and should not give rise to a callow cynicism. But in case of the gap between the vivid New World dream and its actual translation, the contradictions are so numerous and the achievements so spotty and smirched that they almost defy any systematic treatment.

By and large, this is the problem that I have encountered in being a part of the Institution of Vocational Rehabilitation. Throughout the sixteen years that I have been intimately associated with it, first as director of a graduate training program at one of our eastern institutions, and for nearly fifteen years as State Director of the Connecticut program, I have been appalled by the gap between its ideally based pronouncements and its system of delivery.

In order to set the record straight and put this conference in its proper historical perspective so that we all can realize how far we have come since the time when the State-Federal program of Vocational Rehabilitation for culturally handicapped or socio-economically disadvantaged was nil, I wish to inform you that it was at a national conference in 1963 of State directors of vocational rehabilitation, university coordinators of graduate training programs, and Federal officials from the office of Vocational Rehabilitation, convening at Miami Beach, that I nearly broke up the conference when I issued a statement calling for an amendment to our basic Vocational Rehabilitation Act of 1954 so that the Blacks and other culturally and/or socio-economically disadvantaged people could be eligible for vocational rehabilitation services. At that time I was thrown off the committee of training and banished to the doghouse but in 1965 and again in 1968 my confrontation and demands paid off for the U.S. Congress did pass such amendments. Of course it goes without saying these were not named the Jim Peters amendments, but the seeds for them were sown right here in the great State of Florida and your project "STAR" is a viable witness to this "acorn" which, if I read the tea leaves properly, will someday in the not too distant future sprout into a giant Oak. For those of us who still bear battle scars of the great movement for civil rights during the fifties and sixties, we remember that it was not just a "Black revolt" but a "Black-white revolution" of all good people from the north, south, east and west. A revolt by people who were right in the only place where right and might resides, their hearts—the human heart. Now, by getting us together in a common cause by working through the established institutions is not "copping out" of the revolution that was won, but merely good and wise business. The order of the day in dealing with the U.S. Government is business, characterized by responsibility and accountability. This has always been the case since the founding of this great nation. To quote Mumford again:

> In the United States this contradiction between ideal aim and act characterized the westward march of the pioneer: one sees it even in the career of Audubon, a spirit deeply enamored of the wilderness, devoting his whole life to observing and depicting the birds and mammals of North America—but almost wrecking these intentions by sinking all his working capital into a steam sawmill, a premature mechanical enterprise that landed him into bankruptcy. The very immigrants who turned their backs to the seaboard settlements in search of independence and freedom, not merely demanded the active aid of the central government in establishing canals, highroads, and railroads; but called upon national troops to protect their settlements and to extrude, appropriate, and when resisted, exterminate the aborigines who stood in their path. What were the Indian 'reservations' but early concentration camps?

What are our urban ghettos but modern concentration camps? What are our ways of thinking, eating and living only black or white, but the establishment's way of keeping us from joining up. I have but one proposal to offer and that is, vocational rehabilitation for the disadvantaged.

(2) The goals of insight and self-knowledge, though desirable, are often unnecessary in effecting behavioral change in the disadvantaged client.

(3) It is improper for the counselor to be overly invested in any one technique for working with the disadvantaged.

(4) It is necessary for the counselor to control his compelling desire for elaborate diagnostics, with its inferences about underlying dynamics (the "graduate student syndrome") and to stick to specific behaviors relating to increasing the client's employability.

(5) The medical model, involving symptomatic treatment and an authority—dependent relationship, is proving to be ineffective with this type of client.

(6) Counselors should try other role models for the client-counselor relationship, such as that of an advocate, friend, peer, etc.

(7) It is sometimes but not always necessary that family pathology be remedied for the disadvantaged client to become employable.

(8) It is necessary for the counselor to get out of the office; follow-up on the job site is particularly important.

(9) Intensive outreach, as exemplified by Employment Service and other special rehabilitation projects, is necessary in order to find appropriate clients.

(10) Personal contact, primarily through the use of trained, indigenous workers in the homes, hangouts and streets of poverty areas can provide the initial components for building the bridge between the rehabilitation agency and the disadvantaged.

(11) Studies should be made on the process of delivery systems in order to reduce dropouts and increase effectiveness of service.

(12) Greater attention should be paid to the effect of the client's environmental setting and its effect upon his behavior.

(13) Some strategies to alter the client's environment, including the attitudes of significant others, should be explored.

(14) An examination of current attitudes, operations and implicit values should be done with regard to the culturally disadvantaged.

Vocational Rehabilitation and its Relevancy to Minority Groups

The Vocational Rehabilitation Program which exists in each state bears no identical format. This is due to the condition that, by the nature of our form of government, the Federal Government cannot dictate to the states in regard to the particular programs which are carried out by the states. Of course, by providing funds for certain programs, the Federal Government can in reality coerce a state government into providing a particular program; and as long as the demands made by the Federal Government are within the limitations of the constitution, a state government can be encouraged to follow a model established in a particular area. This is exactly the situation in regard to vocational rehabilitation. The Vocational Rehabilitation Administration in Washington, which is an arm of the Department of Health, Education, and Welfare, provides funds to the states for certain programs on a matching basis. This means that the state is encouraged to provide funds in order to get a substantially greater amount from the Federal Government for the programs which, to a great extent, have been developed and planned for by the Federal Government.

Up until recently, funds were provided by the Federal Government— in some cases on a two-to-one matching basis and, in other cases, funds were provided differentially to states on a per capita basis and in relationship to the wealth of a state. This has been changed recently so that now funds are matched by the Federal Government on an 80% federal and 20% state basis to all states. What does this mean in regard to state-wide planning for a program which involves the placing of Rehabilitation Counselors into situations where they can serve the disadvantaged? Initially it indicates that the state government must provide adequate matching funds to gain the amount of federal funding which is offered. Secondly, it means that the State, through its Division of Vocational Rehabilitation, has to decide a greater proportion of these funds will be spent to meet the vocational rehabilitation needs of the disadvantaged.

In general, there are two types of administrative units operating at the state agency level. The first is a department or commission of vocational rehabilitation. The chief administrator is responsible directly to the Governor of the State. The second type is a division or bureau. The head or director reports to the Governor and/or to the State Board of Education. There is, of course, less autonomy in the division or bureau structure. These differences are discerned in Figure 1.

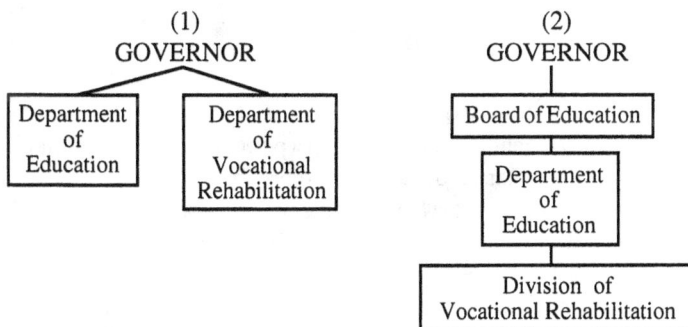

Figure 1: Types of State Administration in Vocation Rehabilitation

The important condition is not that one type is better than the other, but that the particular administrative unit operating in the state has sufficient autonomy for effective functioning, for controlling the essential funds, and for initiating new programs. One of the most negative characteristics relative to the introducing of a new concept, such as establishing a rehabilitation counselor for work with the disadvantaged, is bureaucratic rigidity and inertia. There is a great need for cooperation and understanding of the roles which all of the professional members are to play in order to be most helpful to, for example, clients who are black.

Objectives in Statewide Planning.

Before any new program is initiated, specific objectives must be stated so that a vocational rehabilitation project with emphasis on any aspect of helping individuals can be successfully implemented. Among these objectives are the following:

(1)To identify the handicapped or disadvantaged individuals who are in need of vocational rehabilitation services by interviewing, testing, evaluating, etc. This objective more specifically refers to those individuals who are in school or in the community and who need the closer contact which a counselor can provide. Once the identification process is completed, then planning can proceed.

(2)To formulate a plan which will include the particular goals of a specific group in the community. This objective further encompasses the staff required, along with the funds necessary, for realization of those goals, and workshops, and center for the rehabilitation process.

(3)To identify the resources and services of vocational rehabilitation which will be required at some future time for achieving specific or general goals, for example, various research centers or rehabilitation and demonstration grants may be feasible for survey or evaluative purposes. This can be accomplished through special project funding.

Planning for a Specific Area

To initiate a rehabilitation program in a particular area or community first calls for acceptance by the Governor, the political parties, the Department of Education, the labor unions (who will want to integrate the program with their apprenticeship and employment procedures), representatives of the disadvantaged group or groups, such as the Urban League, and representatives of some of the major employment industrial concerns in the state, such as the Manufacturer's Association and the Chamber of Commerce. It is important that the major agencies, which are in some way involved with the employment of the disadvantaged, are approached in a systematic fashion.

One of the most functional ways of implementing this objective would be for the Governor of the state to name an advisory committee. For example, the State of Connecticut had a Citizen's Advisory Committee for Vocational Rehabilitation, which was concerned with state-wide planning. Its findings and recommendations were very helpful in keeping the program moving in a positive fashion during a period of tight money, both federal and state. This same committee could, in turn, be vested with the responsibility for accumulating and distributing knowledge about the proposed program and for gaining acceptance by the groups listed above and work as an advocate for the disadvantaged. The members of this committee would be vested with planning of extensive responsibility and accountability by the state agency. Not only would the members have to convince the legislature to appropriate funds in order to gain full matching of federal funding, in addition they would have the responsibility for encouraging the Division of Vocational Rehabilitation, or the Commission, to budget appropriate funds for the initiation of the rehabilitation programs for the disadvantaged. The members may have to form a lobbying committee in order to bring such a process into fruition.

The public also has to be informed as to the general nature of the venture. For example, the question may be raised as to the difference between vocational rehabilitation and vocational education; or the difference between an apprenticeship in a trade and a person who is becoming an apprentice under a Vocational Rehabilitation program. The public, industry, and public education all have to know the difference. Each has to be assured that this new venture is not an overlapping or redundant procedure. In addition, each has to be reassured that the procedures proposed would help many disadvantaged people who need help. However, in a state where Vocational Rehabilitation is neither under the Department of Education nor exists as a separate commission, need for careful planning at the state level is obvious. The delineation and recognition of those individuals who will be involved in such a program has to take place.

As in most states, the State of Connecticut has several district offices where an important question, which initially had to be answered, was whether disadvantaged persons who qualified should be served through district offices or whether a separate administrative system coming directly form the state level should furnish rehabilitation counseling to these people through some other mechanism. The answer to this question deals not only with administrative protocol, but also with fiscal procedures, as service funds will have to be channeled to the rehabilitation counselor in the district office. In addition, since he should be supervised, in all probability the distance to a local district office will in some respects determine whether or not he should be supervised by that office. It might be possible to set up a person in the Central DVR office who would have authority over all counselors with and for the disadvantaged located throughout the state; or, rehabilitation counselors in each district office could be responsible for this work to the authority of a district supervisor or director located in the office where he works. It was our experience in the Bridgeport Project for the disadvantaged that the in-school rehabilitation counselor should be under the jurisdiction of the local supervisor. The services and the service funds emanated from this local office. Our reasons for this position were many. For example, it was logical that some of the clients who were referred to the school rehabilitation counselor were not able to be serviced by him, due to their unique disability. Such clients were referred easily from one rehabilitation counselor to another working for the same supervisor, boss, etc. In addition, any procedure which is preventing the processing of a client is easily resolved when the school rehabilitation counselor is a field representative with ties to the district office.

Another question to be answered at the state-wide level is how rapidly a special program for the disadvantaged should develop. For example, how many rehabilitation counselors will be furnished the program in the first year? A related question deals with the amount of service funds which will be available to these rehabilitation counselors each year as their role expands. In the city of Bridgeport, the number of disadvantaged students who were referred and who qualified under the disability codes was so great that a limit had to be set on the amount of service funds which could be utilized, otherwise it would have infringed upon the regular rehabilitation program offered through the district office.

In the State of Connecticut an objective of the administration is to place a rehabilitation counselor in every high school having an enrollment of one thousand or more. These counselors will be available to a large number of disadvantaged young people and could be very helpful in assisting them with their vocational plans. A second objective is to serve three or more smaller high schools in towns bordering one another which do not have an enrollment far greater than 600. This will take care of the rural disadvantaged and migrant workers. Arrangements and planning at the state level are, to a great extent, more easily accomplished than planning within the local community. This is due to the greater number of agencies which must be contacted and encouraged to accept this new idea in the local community. The great number of high schools which exist in the State of Connecticut precluded the inclusion of a representative from each city or town serving on, for example, the Citizen's Advisory Committee. While this procedure would benefit a local planning group, it would make the State Advisory Group much too large and cumbersome. Hence, after the Administration devised a state-wide plan, which delineates how specific cities and towns would be classified, the next step was for a representative of the State agency to visit the local Administration Officer in the town and discuss the matter with the Superintendent of Schools, as well as with the Administrator of the local community, such as the Mayor or First Selectman. The services and funds which the rehabilitation counselor brings with him obviously are welcomed in any city or school as long as the handicapped children can benefit. Although the Mayor and the Superintendent of Schools are willing to meet with the Rehabilitation Counselor or a representative of the Vocational Rehabilitation Program, there are many problems which have to be solved before the Vocational Rehabilitation Counselor will be able to function in the border community. If the planning at the State level has been completed in a careful manner, then planning at the local community level will follow easily and naturally.

The Citizens' Advisory Committee should be available to monitor and advise D.V.R. in regard to its present program and future plans. Having a Citizens' Advisory Committee, which maintains a constant liaison to the State Government, assures that people are being served as well as the industries which will eventually employ them.

Perhaps it will be found necessary to create an inter-divisional technical committee within the Division of Vocational Rehabilitation in order to maintain the lines of communication among the State Office of Vocational Rehabilitation, the district office, and the school rehabilitation counselor. Providing for and maintaining the understanding and acceptance of the program by regular D.V.R. personnel is an absolute necessity—for the ongoing success of the program, for its growth and development, and for the ultimate rehabilitation of the disadvantaged.

Are there any rehabilitation agencies run and operated by Black people with BVR support?

(1)Paying for client services through Black designed and implemented programs in their own communities.

(2)How effective are white counselors with Black clients;

    A.statement of problems

    B.training programs to eliminate counseling error with minorities—other solutions.

(3)Placement problems with Black clients as compared with whites.

(4)Is the organization of a BVR. suited to handle special problems arising in minority communities?

(5)Any special grants of money to predominate Black rehabilitation agencies, if any:

Has the State been instrumental in helping people get agencies started in minority communities?

Administrative Organization of the Division of Vocation Rehabilitation

In order to understand and appreciate the working of the official state agency for rehabilitating handicapped people, one should become acquainted with its organizational structure. This agency has both federal and state laws to conform to, as well as live with, but here we concern ourselves only with Connecticut's general statutes for they follow federal statutes in most instances. This is important so that Blacks and other minorities can learn where the power is and can influence this power to their advantage. This is good for the entire community.

Designation of State Agency

(a)The State Board of Education which administers vocational education in the State is designated as the sole agency to administer the vocational rehabilitation program. The State legislature has given legal authority for such designation, which is contained in Sections 10-100 through 10-108 of the General Statutes, Revision of 1958, as amended.

(b)Section 10-101 of the General Statutes was repealed by PA 91 of the February special session of 1965 of the General Assembly and the following substituted in lieu thereof: The State Board of Education shall maintain a Vocational Rehabilitation (unit) Division and shall disburse all funds provided for such rehabilitation, except for services to the blind. Said Board shall appoint and subject to the provisions of Section 4-40, fix the compensation of such persons as may be necessary to administer the provisions of Sections 10-100 to 10-108, inclusive, and may, within said (unit) division, create such sections as will facilitate such administration, including a disability determinations section for which one-hundred percent federal funds may be accepted for the operation of such section in conformity with applicable state and federal regulations.

Responsibility of State Agency

All decisions affecting the eligibility of clients, or the nature and scope of vocational rehabilitation services to be provided, will be made by the State Vocational Rehabilitation Agency, and this responsibility will not be delegated to any other agency or individual not of the agency stuff.

Organization of State Agency

The State Vocational Rehabilitation Agency maintains a central or administrative office with bureaus, and an administrative services section, as a (unit) Division of the State Department of Education in Hartford, the capitol of Connecticut, as well as a system of district and local offices, strategically located throughout the state.

The central office and administrative service section, through its bureaus, functions to provide direction, supervision, coordination and overall fiscal management of the rehabilitation program. In addition, professional and technical information, research and consultative services are made available to district and local offices.

The system of district and local offices functions to locate, investigate, evaluate, counsel, provide and supervise rehabilitation services to handicapped individuals found to be eligible for needed services. Local offices, under the supervision of a district office, are established in suitable locations for the purpose of integrating the state agency program more effectively into community organization and participation.

Executive direction and coordination stems from the Director of the state agency, through the Chief of the Bureau of Vocational Rehabilitation Services, to District Directors and Counselors. While each member of the professional staff is responsible to provide public information and program interpretation, the Consultant for In-Service Training and Public Information functions to furnish leadership in promoting and coordinating these activities; in addition, this staff member is the editor of the news bulletin published by the Division of Vocational Rehabilitation. This same staff member is responsible also for guidance, training and placement activities of the agency program and maintains consultative services to district and local office staffs. The Counselor is responsible for counseling of clients and for developing plans with them for the provision of needed services.

Physical restoration services are an integral part of the state agency program and are provided only on the recommendation of competent medical opinion. The medical responsibility for recommendation of physical restoration services rests primarily with medical consultants attached on a part-time basis to each district office and to the larger local offices. These consultants refer problem situations to the Chief Medical Officer who serves as the State agency's Medical Administrative Consultant. In addition, the Chief of the Bureau of Vocational Rehabilitation Services also serves as Supervisor of Physical Restoration, and in this capacity works closely with the staffs of district and local offices, and with the Administrative and District Medical Consultants with respect to the provision of physical restoration services.

The Division, through its Bureau of Disability Determination, is the agency delegated to carry out the contract for making disability determinations on behalf of the Social Security Administration.

The Chief of the Bureau of Community and Institutional Services will be responsible for planning concerned with rehabilitation facilities including cooperative programs. He will secure adequate information concerning such programs to be given to the staff through the Consultant on In-Service Training.

It will be the policy of the State agency to secure consultative services for special disability groups from proper sources. Where necessary, the Division Director and appropriate staff members will furnish leadership in specialized programs as required. (For example, in homebound programs, etc.)

The District Director is responsible to the Director through the Chief of the Bureau of Vocational Rehabilitation Services, for the operation and administration of a district office and of the local offices established within the area served by the district office. The District Director plans, directs and supervises the rehabilitation program within the district; advises counselors in respect to planning and scheduling of work, selection of cases, methods of handling cases and availability of services to meet applicant needs, integrates all services necessary for successful rehabilitation of disabled individuals; reviews flow sheets and other case load control devises; supervises staff in carrying out sound individual rehabilitation plans; plan and operates the district office budget and is responsible for maintenance of accurate fiscal records of the transactions within the district office area.

Under the Leadership of the administrative office, research will be conducted and statistics maintained on various phases of program operation. This will include necessary information for purposes of program planning, program revision or improvement, budgeting, and other necessary research in connection with special studies.

The budget of the State agency is prepared in the administrative office with the cooperation of the District Directors. Fiscal supervision is maintained in the administrative office, where the Administrative Service Officer plans, organizes and implements fiscal and other general business activities of the agency in consultation with the agency head and representatives of the central state agencies.

Local Rehabilitation Agencies
No part of the State agency program is administered by a local agency.

State Director
The chief administrative head of the Division is the Director who is responsible to the Secretary of the State Board of Education. Executive direction of the bureaus and sub-sections are coordinated by him with the assistance of bureau chiefs and other central office administrative aides and consultants. The responsibilities of the Division Director are discharged within the confines of state and federal regulations. Certain specific tasks are necessarily and properly delegated to subordinates, but the final responsibility for decision and the power of approval and review of actions of subordinates remains with him. The Director may properly be responsive to the suggestions and information of his subordinates but only he may decide what goals should established for the Division, for responsibility of realizing them is his.

The Director of the State agency devotes full time and effort to the program of the Division of Vocational Rehabilitation. This consists of the various bureaus and subdivisions indicated below.

Chief of the Bureau of Vocational Rehabilitation Services
The Chief of the Bureau of Vocational Rehabilitation Services is responsible to the Division Director for:

(a) The realization of the specific program goals of the Division with respect to the numbers and kinds of cases rehabilitated and with respect to the manner and quality of their rehabilitation.

(b) The organization, administration and disposition of the staff made available to him so as to make them most effective in the realization of the Division program goals.

(c) Planning and preparing for the manpower needs of the rehabilitation service. This process should include allocating duties among members of the staff in such a way that those staff members for whom promotion is a possibility should be given the opportunity and encouragement to undertake formal training to fit them for promotion and should be given the opportunity for professional and administrative experience that will likewise fit them for promotion. This should apply not only to positions specifically designated as training positions but also to other positions.

(d) The establishment and maintenance of a system for ensuring that high professional standards of a case-work are maintained by the counseling staff.

(e) The preparation, publication and necessary amendment of a manual of case-work practices for counselors and area supervisors.

(f) The assessment of the incidence of disability by class and the estimation of future probable case loads by geographical distribution, disability, and number and, in conjunction with the Administrative Service Officer and others, for preparing projections of the need for funds for case services and rehabilitation counseling personnel.

(g) The assessment of the present and probably future opportunities for the placement of the rehabilitated, and acting to anticipate the effect of changes in placement opportunities and patterns of employment upon the placement of the rehabilitated.

(h) Acting and recommending action to the staff and to the Division Director to reduce restrictions on the employment of the rehabilitated and to widen and increase their opportunities for employment.

(i) Informing the staff of new developments in rehabilitation techniques that are applicable to the program, and acting to encourage the use of such developments in technique when they would further the attainment of the goals of the Division.

(j) The communication of the relevant ultimate and operating goals of the Division to the members of the staff.

(k) Encouraging the members of the staff to play an active role in communicating the achievements and goals of the Division to the General public and to organizations both within and without the rehabilitation field, and for seeking the aid of the Consultant on In-Service Training and Public Information to this end.

(l) Ensuring, by means including an active in-service training program, that the state of knowledge and level of training of the professional staff is such as to best further the attainment of the goals of the Division and for seeking the aid of the Consultant on In-Service Training and Public Information to this end.

(m) Informing the Division Director of the activities and achievements of the staff and of the degree to which the established goals of the Division are being achieved.

Chief of the Bureau of Disability Determination

The Chief of the Bureau of Disability Determination is responsible to the Division Director for:

(a) The establishment and implementation of procedures to fulfill the Division's responsibility to make disability determinations on behalf of the Secretary of Health, Education, and Welfare for the Social Security Administration.

(b) The organization and administration of program and staff so as to most effectively achieve the goals of the Division and the Social Security Administration.

(c) The formulation and implementation of staff development and training of disability adjudication staff, in coordination with the Division's training program.

(d) The projection and justification of funds for budgetary purposes, as well as the determination of staffing needs.

(e) The review and transmission of statistical case data to federal and state authorities.

(f) The development and maintenance of effective methods of the appraisal of vocational rehabilitation potential in connection with referral and selection of Social Security disability applicants for rehabilitation services.

(g) The effective use and development of rehabilitation facilities including psychological, medical and vocational areas in coordination with the Division.

(h) The carrying out of Federal regulations, procedures and laws governing the program. This includes liaison activities with local, regional and national Social Security offices. Reciprocal medical evaluation services between states are provided for those applicants moving outside of Connecticut. Special evaluation services are likewise provided to the Federal Bureau of Hearings and Appeals.

(i) The establishment of plans and systems of operational procedures designed to most efficiently execute the processing of disability claims.

(j) The fostering of public program understanding by utilization of staff in effective contacts with agencies and professional groups.

(k) The overall supervision of a staff of professional, medical and secretarial personnel who function in the adjudication process.

Chief of Bureau of Community and Institutional Services

The Chief of Bureau of Community and Institutional Services is responsible to the Division Director for:

(a) Developing a detailed forecast of needed facilities in response to the projections of future probable case load prepared by the Chief of Rehabilitation Services.

(b) Making and maintaining a detailed inventory of rehabilitation facilities available to the Division.

(c) Planning and promoting the development of rehabilitation facilities in response to the program needs of the Division, and regularly informing the Division Director of the extent to which the present and future facility needs are being or are likely to be met.

(d) Planning and negotiating contracts for the supply of services with private and state rehabilitation agencies, with the aid and counsel of the Administrative Service Officer in the matter of price.

(e) Administering contracts negotiated in (d) above, including the control of quality of service, and ensuring conformance with Division policies and ensuring consistency with Division goals, except where the contracts involve the continued deployment within the contracting agency of members of the Division staff.

(f) Negotiating cooperative programs with other state and municipal agencies.

(g) Administering cooperative programs negotiated in (f) above in similar manner to the administration of contracts for service and with similar limitations.

(h) Informing the Division Director and other members of the staff of new developments in rehabilitation techniques that are available in Connecticut, or ought to be available in Connecticut.

(i) To extend and improve vocational rehabilitation services to the disabled person, with special emphasis on the severely disabled. The Chief of the Bureau of Community and Institutional Services will act as liaison between sheltered workshops and the Rehabilitation Division and will act as a consultant to public and private organizations planning to establish sheltered workshops and rehabilitation facilities in Connecticut.

New workshops for the disabled are being established in various parts of the State. Rapid expansion of existing workshops is taking place. Important in the expansion of services for the severely disabled has been the initiation of new types of services in many workshops. These new services show promise of helping severely disabled clients for whom we have been able to accomplish to little to often.

The addition of a workshop coordinator will allow the Rehabilitation Division to secure more adequate information as to the types of service available, costs, procedures, etc. This information can be transmitted to counselors through the Consultant on In-Service Training at an early date to insure better services for rehabilitation clients.

The Rehabilitation Division has been helpful in the development of the Connecticut Workshop Association. All operating workshops are now members or are in the process of becoming members. The Association has expressed a need for an individual to coordinate its activities with the Rehabilitation Division and to provide information regarding new procedures in workshops throughout the country.

Consultation with community groups and public and private agencies and officials is necessary if we are to aid in the establishment of workshops where there is a definite need.

This program of coordination of rehabilitation facilities and sheltered workshop activities with the Vocational Rehabilitation program will be under the direction of the Chief of the Bureau of Community and Institutional Services, His specific duties will be:

(1) Consult with and advise community groups, public and private agencies and officials on the establishment and operation of sheltered workshops.

(2) Evaluate and examine proposals and plans for the establishment of workshops.

(3) Develop agreements regarding the purchase of workshop services and give technical advice in relation to the establishment of fee schedules for these workshop services.

(4) Provide assistance in any advisory capacity to workshops attempting to work toward the standards set up by the National and State associations.

(5) Consult with workshop administrators regarding the development of Public Relations Programs in the community. These programs to be coordinated with the program of the Division, which is the responsibility of the Consultant on In-Service Training and Public Information.

(6) Provide assistance to workshops in establishing programs for personal adjustment, work evaluation, work conditioning, and work tryout job training.

(7) Provide assistance to workshops on such matters as work layout production, production contracts and other similar operations.

(8) Develop written agreements for projects involving grants of State and Federal funds to workshops, including the establishment and maintenance of adequate records and accounts to assure that expenditures are in accord with the grant award and to provide for prior approval when a material change in the scope of the project or its operation is contemplated.

(9) Make inspection at regular intervals to assure that the actual program of services and utilization of equipment provided are as agreed in the approved project application.

(10) Initiate surveys and reviews of the progress in workshops, prepare and submit regular reports of the needs and trends in workshop development.

(11) Consult with administrators of workshops with respect to establishing and maintaining standards of services for the rehabilitation of Division clients.

Administrative Service officer

The Administrative Service Officer is responsible to the Division Director for:

(a) The formulation of detailed fiscal and personnel policies, systems, and procedures within the constraints of Departmental, State and Federal regulations.

(b) The development of annual budgets and of longer term financial plans in response to the projections of program needs made by the Chief of the Bureau of Vocational Rehabilitation Services and the Chief of the Bureau of Community and Institutional Services.

(c) The preparation of cost estimates in response to specific program proposals made by the Chief of the Bureau of Community and Institutional Services or the Chief of the Bureau of Vocational Rehabilitation Services or the Division Director.

(d) The preparation of monthly, quarterly and other fiscal and statistical reports, projections of income and expenditures and other necessary short-term financial plans for the Division Director.

(e) The interpretation of these periodic and special reports for the staff, and the recommendation of actions to be taken in response to the information they afford.

(f) The maintenance of such Division statistical and fiscal records as are not maintained by the Division of Administration and are not maintained in the Field offices.

(g) The maintenance of such personnel records for the Division as are not maintained by the Division of Administration for the Division, and for monitoring and supervising the program of performance evaluation that is established for the Division. The establishment of procedures for qualifying vendors used by the Division, and the implementation of those procedures established, as necessary.

(h) Establishing and maintaining a numerically or otherwise encoded catalog of all qualified vendors and the services supplied by them, including the prices and conditions of such services.

(i) Negotiating prices for services purchased by the Division, directly with the vendor, or through the appropriate agency of the State.

(j) The post-auditing of requisitions for rehabilitation services issued by counselors and the initiation of actions to correct errors discovered.

(k) The preparation and authorization of requisitions for consumable stores and equipment.

In addition to the above, the Administrative Service Officer is responsible for planning, organizing and business management functions involving the making of important administrative decisions on the activities of the agency; assists the agency head in formulating and is responsible for implementing policy in the fiscal, office services and other general business activities of the agency; directs the budgetary and fiscal control programs; consults with Bureau supervisors on administrative problems and procedures and assists in developing and instituting improvements; directs the operation of the accounting system and the preparation of detailed financial statements and statistical reports; coordinates the requisitioning and use of supplies and equipment to insure efficient material control; directs the storage of supplies and inventory control; confers on the storage of supplies and inventory control; confers on problems of auditing, accounting, budgeting, purchasing and personnel with representative of central State agencies; makes special administrative studies; prepares reports and dictates correspondence; at institutions is responsible for the general operation and inspection of the grounds, service facilities and buildings to insure efficient and economical service and repair and confers with unit supervisor on problems of operation and management.

Consultant for In-Service Training and Public Information

The Consultant for In-Service Training and Public Information is responsible to the Division for:

(a) Ascertaining, in conjunction with the Bureau Chiefs and the members of their staffs, the present in-service and off-duty training needs of the professional and clerical staffs and their future needs in the light of projected program developments and projected manpower needs.

(b) Planning, developing and executing a program of in-service training for the professional staff including:

(1) Promoting the development of needed training courses at educational facilities both in Connecticut and elsewhere that are available to the members of the staff.

(2) Arranging and enabling the attendance of members of the staff at the courses so developed.

(3) Arranging individual and group training programs within the Division where such training would be suitable.

(4) Promoting and facilitating the supply of needed instructional and technical material to the members of the staff in response to their needs and/or at the request of the Chief of the Bureau of Vocational Rehabilitation Services, the Chief of the Bureau of Disability Determination or the Chief of the Bureau of Community and Institutional Services.

With the rapid development of workshops, new programs, new objectives, new techniques and a variety of nomenclature, close liaison and increased communications are needed in order to keep Rehabilitation Division counselors abreast of changing conditions.

(c) Planning, developing and executing a program of public information, including:

(1) The preparation and publishing of a periodic newsletter concerned with events of rehabilitation interest for distribution to members of the staff and to interested persons and organizations outside the Division.

(2) The preparation and dissemination to the staff of publicity material such as outline speeches and audio-visual material about rehabilitation subjects in anticipation of general and particular opportunities for public information use of the staff.

(3) The coaching and support of members of the staff in preparation for specific occasions for public information.

(4) Reviewing and assessing the effectiveness of particular efforts of public information with the members of staff concerned and for the information of other members of the staff.

(5) The seeking out of opportunities for informing the public and the encouragement of members of the staff in responding to such opportunities.

(6) In conjunction with other staff members, identifying and structuring relations with other public and private agencies whose cooperation will facilitate the attainment of the goals of the agency.

𝕮

CHAPTER NINETEEN

REHABILITATION AND THE LAW— CONFIDENTIALITY

James S. Peters, II, Ph.D.
Division of Vocational Rehabilitation
Connecticut State Department of Education
Hartford, Connecticut

It is a pleasure for me to speak on "Rehabilitation and the Law," with emphasis on Confidentiality. Vocational rehabilitation, as conceived during the early 1920s by the Congress and various State legislatures, is steeped in legalistic and moral imperatives as to this aspect of its responsibility to clients and the citizenry. We state vocational rehabilitation workers live with these legal and moral problems each day as we attempt to carry out the mandate of the Congress. I only need to cite the preamble to our recently enacted Act, Public Law 93-112 of the 93rd Congress:

> An Act to replace the Vocational Rehabilitation Act, to extend and revise the authorization of grants to States for vocational rehabilitation services, with special emphasis on services to those with the most severe handicaps, to expand special Federal responsibilities and research and training programs with respect to handicapped individuals within the Department of Health, Education, and Welfare, and for other purposes.

The Act is very comprehensive as legally enacted by the Senate and House of Representatives of the United States of America in Congress assembled, and signed by the President. There are three titles to the Act:

Paper given as Panel Member, Northeast Region, National Rehabilitation Association, Bretton Woods, New Hampshire, May 30, 1974.

Title I—Vocational Rehabilitation Services
    Part A—General Provisions
    Part B—Basic Vocational Rehabilitation Services
    Part C—Innovation and Expansion Grants
    Part D—Comprehensive Service Needs
Title II—Research and Training
Title IV—Administration and Program and Project Evaluation
Title V—Miscellaneous

It is in Section 2 of the Act that we derive its function. This section sets forth the "Declaration of Purpose" and I quote:

> The purpose of this Act is to provide a statutory basis for the Rehabilitation Services Administration, and to authorize programs to—
> (1) develop and implement comprehensive and continuing State plans for meeting the current and future needs for providing vocational rehabilitation services to handicapped individuals and to provide such services for the benefit of such individuals, serving first those with the most severe handicaps, so that they may prepare for and engage in gainful employment;
> (2) evaluate the rehabilitation potential of handicapped individual;
> (3) conduct a study to develop methods of providing rehabilitation services to meet the current and future needs of handicapped individuals for whom a vocational goal is not possible or feasible so that they may improve their ability to live with greater independence and self-sufficiency;
> (4) assist in the construction and improvement of rehabilitation facilities;
> (5) develop new and innovative methods of applying the most advanced medical technology, scientific achievement, and psychological and social knowledge to solve rehabilitation problems and develop new and innovative methods of providing rehabilitation services to handicapped individuals through research, special projects, and demonstrations;
> (6) initiate and expand services to groups of handicapped individuals (including those who are homebound

or institutionalized) who have been underserved in the past;

(7)conduct various studies and experiments to focus on long neglected problem areas;

(8)promote and expand employment opportunities in the public and private sectors for handicapped individuals and to place such individuals in employment;

(9)establish client assistance pilot projects;

(10)provide assistance for the purposes of increasing the number of rehabilitation personnel and increasing their skills through training; and

(11)evaluate existing approaches to architectural and transportation barriers confronting handicapped individuals, develop new approaches, enforce statutory and regulatory standards and requirements regarding barrier-free construction of public facilities and study and develop solutions to existing architectural and transportation barriers impeding handicapped individuals.

The soon to be released Federal regulations of the Act, Section 401.44 *Confidential Information,* is as follows:

(a)The State plan shall provide that the State agency will adopt such regulations as are necessary to assure that:

(1)All information as to personal facts given or made available to the State agency, its representatives, or its employees, in the course of the administration of the vocational rehabilitation program, including lists of names and addresses and records of agency evaluation, shall be held to be confidential.

(2)The use of such information and records shall be limited to purposes directly connected with the administration of the vocational rehabilitation program and shall not be disclosed, directly or indirectly, other than in the administration thereof, unless the consent of the client to such release has been obtained whether expressly or by necessary implication, or the client expressly requests the information and records for purposes in connection with any proceeding or action for benefits or damages, including any proceeding for action against any public agency, in which case the State agency shall release, pursuant to such request, such information and records as are relevant to the needs of the client. Release of pertinent information to employers in connection with the placement of the client may be considered as release of information in connection with the administration of the vocational rehabilitation program. Such information may, however, be released to welfare agencies or other programs from which the client has requested certain services under circumstances from which his consent may be presumed, provided such agencies have adopted regulations which will assure that the information will be used only for the purposes for which it is provided. Such information will be released to an organization or individual engaged in research only for purposes directly connected with the administration of the State vocational rehabilitation program and only if the organization or individual furnished satisfactory assurance that the information will be used only for the purpose for which it is provided; that it will not be released to persons not connected with the study of consideration; and that the final product of the research will not reveal any information that may serve to identify any person about whom information has been obtained through the State agency, without written consent of such person and the State agency.

(3)All such information is the property of the State agency.

(b)The State plan shall further provide that the State agency will adopt such procedures and standards as are necessary to:

(1)Give effect to these regulations; and

(2)Assure that all rehabilitation applicants, clients and interested persons will be informed as to the confidentiality of vocational rehabilitation information.

Under Section 15.0 of Connecticut State Plan for Vocational Rehabilitation Services, is found Confidential Information. It reads as follows:

The Division of Vocational Rehabilitation has adopted regulations and policies to assure that:

(1)All information as to personal facts given or made

available to the state agency, its representatives, or its employees, in the course of administration of the vocational rehabilitation program, including lists of names and addresses and records of agency evaluation, will be held to be confidential.

(2)The use of such information and records will be limited to purposes directly connected with the administration of the vocational rehabilitation program and may not be disclosed, directly or indirectly, other than in the administration thereof, unless the consent of the client to such release has been obtained either expressly or by necessary implication. Release of information to employers in connection with the placement of the client may be considered as release of information in connection with the administration of the vocational rehabilitation program. Such information may, however, be released to welfare agencies or programs from which the client has requested certain services under circumstances from which his consent may be presumed, provided such agencies have adopted regulations which will assure that the information will be held confidential, and can assure that the information will be used only for the purpose for which it is provided. Such information will be released to an organization or individual engaged in research only for purposes directly connected with the administration of the State Vocational Rehabilitation Program (including research for the development of new knowledge or techniques which would be useful in the administration of the program) and only if the organization or individual furnishes satisfactory assurance that the information will be used only for the purpose for which it is provided; that it will not be released to persons not connected with the study under consideration; and that the final product of the research will not reveal any information that may serve to identify any person about whom information has been obtained through the state agency without written consent of such person and the state agency.

(3)All such information is the property of the state agency and may be used only in accordance with the agency's regulations.

The Division of Vocational Rehabilitation has adopted standards and operating procedures necessary to: (1) give effect to its regulations; (2) assure that all rehabilitation clients and interested persons will be informed as to the confidentiality of vocational rehabilitation information; (3) assure the adoption of such office practice and the availability of such office facilities and equipment as will assure the adequate protection of the confidentiality of such records.

Under the "Connecticut Right to Know Law" is this information:

Sec. 1-19. Access to public records. Except as otherwise provided by any federal or state statute or regulation, all records made, maintained or kept on file by any executive, administrative, legislative or judicial body, agency, commission or official of the state, or any political subdivision thereof, whether or not such records are required by any law or by any rule or regulation, shall be public records and every resident of the state shall have the right to inspect or copy such records sat such reasonable time as may be determined by the custodian thereof. Each such executive, administrative, legislative and judicial body, agency, commission or official shall keep and maintain all public records in his custody at his regular office or place of business in an accessible place and, if there is no such office or place of business, the public records pertaining to such body, agency, commission or official shall be kept in the office of the town clerk or the secretary of the state, as the case may be. Any certified record hereunder attested as a true copy by the chief or deputy of such executive, administrative, legislative and judicial body, agency, commission or official shall be competent evidence in any court of this state of the facts contained therein. Each such executive, administrative, legislative and judicial body, agency, commission or official shall make, keep and maintain a record of the proceedings of its meetings. Internal personnel rules and practices of any such body, agency, commission or official, trade secrets and commercial or financial information obtained from the public; inter-agency or intra-agency memoranda or letters dealing solely with matters of law or policy; personnel or medical files and similar files the disclosure of which would constitute an invasion of personal privacy, and investigatory files compiled for law enforcement purposes, except to the extent available by law to a private citizen, shall not be deemed public records for the purposes of this section, provided disclosure pursuant to the provisions of this section shall be required of all records of investigation conducted with respect to any tenement house, lodging house or boarding house as defined in chapter 352, by any municipal building department or housing code inspection department, any local or district health department, or any other department charged with the enforcement of ordinances or laws regulating the erection, construction, alteration, maintenance, sanitation, ventilation or occupancy of such buildings. (1957, P.A. 428, S. 1; 1963, P.A. 260; 1967, P.A. 723, S.1; 1969, P.A. 193; 1971, P.A. 193.)

Ethical standards for Rehabilitation Counselors, prepared by the NRCA Ethics Sub-Committee, and accepted at San Juan, Puerto Rico, September 1972, follow:

A rehabilitation counselor has a commitment to the effective functioning of all human beings; his emphasis is on facilitating the functioning or refunctioning of those persons who are at some disadvantage in the struggle to achieve viable goals. While fulfilling this commitment he interacts with many people, programs, institutions, demands and concepts, and in many different types of relationship. In his endeavors he seeks to enhance the welfare of his clients and of all others whose welfare his professional roles and activities will affect. He recognizes that both action and inaction can be facilitating or debilitating and he accepts the responsibility for his action and inaction.

The acceptable rules of behavior which the rehabilitation counselor himself observes and which he urges his colleagues to observe are in relationships with (1) his client, (2) his client's family, (3) his client's employer or prospective employer, (4) his fellow counselor, (5) his colleagues in other professions, (6) his own employer or supervisor, (7) the community, (8) other programs, agencies and institutions, (9) maintenance of his technical competency, and (10) research. The ethical rules presented here are organized to group specific rules or principles as they cluster about these various relationships.

Counselor—Client

I. The primary obligation of the rehabilitation counselor is to his client. In all his relationships he will protect the client's welfare and will diligently seek to assist the client towards his goals.

A. The rehabilitation counselor will keep confidential any information he acquires concerning the client, the divulgence of which might be inimical to the best interests of the clients.

1. The rehabilitation counselor will persist in claiming the "privileged" status of confidential information concerning his clients in court proceeding.

2. Where there are conflicts between the client's interests and the interests and welfare of the community, the rehabilitation counselor will protect the client, unless by his doing so there is created a real and imminent danger to others.

a. The counselor will try to persuade the client to report knowledge of crimes or planned crimes to the appropriate law enforcement authorities.

b. The client will be warned that information acquired in the counseling relationship might have to be reported in court proceedings; that it might not be possible to withhold the information as "privileged."

3. Where illegal behavior of the client is destructive to himself as well as to the community, the rehabilitation counselor will report such behavior to the appropriate authorities, after advising the client that this must be done.

4. In situations where it is necessary to share information with other in order to advance the rehabilitation goals of the client, consent of the client or his guardian or parent will be secured before release of such information.

a.Only information essential to advancing the goals of the client will be given to others.

b.Only these persons for whom it is essential to have information about the client in order to advance his rehabilitation will be given information.

5. Only such information as the client requires to advance his rehabilitation will be given to him. The counselor will personally give and interpret information to the client that is within the scope of the rehabilitation counseling specialty to develop and establish.

6. Only information essential to advancing the goals of the client will be included in the records kept on the client.

7. Client records will be safeguarded to insure that unauthorized persons shall not have access to them.

a.All nonprofessional persons who mush have access to the client's records will be thoroughly briefed concerning the confidentiality standards to be observed. Compliance with these standards will be continuously monitored by the counselor and will be his responsibility.

b.The counselor will insist on an administrative plan for retirement and destruction of client records that will afford satisfactory protection of the client's future interests and welfare.

❦

CHAPTER TWENTY

REHABILITATION'S GREAT PARTNERSHIP

James S. Peters, II and Seymour J. Mund

"It's a problem, Jim. Can you help?"

"If we work together, we can try to resolve it."

This phone conversation is a common occurrence between the director of the Connecticut Vocational Rehabilitation program and directors of the privately owned and operated nonprofit rehabilitation facilities within the state. This partnership between the public and private sector has been an important part of the rehabilitation scene for over 20 years, and has proven both economical and efficient. It is a positive example of the attitude of cooperation for the betterment of people with handicaps.

This combination of private initiative with matching government money and technical assistance has been a major factor in the expansion of services to disabled people in the State of Connecticut.

In the late 1950's when DVR programs were expanding, the first author was appointed director of the Connecticut Division of Vocational Rehabilitation. At the time, he had the option of developing a program of state-operated rehabilitation facilities or expanding the handful of privately run facilities then in operation. Based on Connecticut's long history of private enterprise and a strong feeling that the private sector has an important role to play in rehabilitation, the director and his staff decided to push for expansion and development of privately run facilities. The one state-operated rehabilitation center in New Haven was closed by the governor during this period of creative state-private-federal effort. The director and his staff noted the emerging role that the workshops and comprehensive rehabilitation centers were playing in vocational rehabilitation and sought to aid them through federal and state financial assistance.

This article was originally printed in the Journal of Rehabilitation, May/June 1976.

In 1954 a nationwide ferment of interest in expanding vocational rehabilitation culminated in the enactment of legislation which greatly broadened the horizon for disabled people and seemed destined to bring the workshop into closer alliance than ever with its sister programs. The system of federal and state financial support then placed in operation reinforced recognition of workshops as an instrument of rehabilitation, and implemented this acknowledgment through the several financial mechanisms enacted to stimulate and expand vocational rehabilitation facilities, including workshops.

Vocational rehabilitation workers, including workshop administrators, had long recognized the need for more substantial support for creating additional workshops and rehabilitation centers for the training of more professional staff members, and for the development and refinement of rehabilitation techniques. In his health message to Congress, January 18, 1954, the President set an eventual yearly goal for the state-federal program of 200,000 rehabilitated persons, as compared to 61,000 rehabilitations in fiscal year 1953. At the same time the President set the stage for the enactment of the present legislative framework, which is designed to help vocational rehabilitation and other nonprofit agencies attack all of these problems.[1]

Written into the Vocational Rehabilitation Act were special programs designed for facilities. These programs include grants for construction and staffing, technical assistance, training, and more recently, the Laird Amendments and third-party funding possibilities. As stated in the law:

"The Secretary is authorized to make grants to public or other nonprofit rehabilitation facilities to pay part of the cost of projects to analyze, improve and increase their professional services to the handicapped, their business management, or any part of their operations affecting their capacity to provide employment and services for the handicapped."[2]

Using the above authorization given at that time, Connecticut DVR established the Bureau of Community and Institutional Services and encouraged the directors of facilities to apply for the available funds. Many did, and the following are examples of how this cooperation was effective:

Example I

A rapidly growing rehabilitation facility found its expansion causing "growing pains" in several aspects of its administrative and operational performances. The prime concerns were in the areas of time study, pricing, and record keeping procedures of the workshop.

The administrator of the facility applied to the Division of Vocational

Rehabilitation for a technical assistance consultation grant, available under the federal rehabilitation law. This grant was approved and provided the funding for an expert in the field, the DVR facilities consultant, to come to the facility, review its practices and problems, and make recommendations.

The consultant found problems in the expected areas. However, he also found other problems directly caused by rapid expansion. He proceeded to offer recommendations to alleviate problems within the original intent of the grant and also in the areas of plant utilization, long-range planning and promotion, and development of the facility.

The facility has implemented these recommendations and has continued its growth in a more systematic and stable way. This has resulted in an increased availability of improved services to handicapped people within the area of this facility.

Example II

A comprehensive rehabilitation facility expanded services over a period of year. The subsequent result was an increasing need to transport more and more disabled clients to and from the facility. The patients and clients who are provided transportation by the rehabilitation facility are persons who have, at the time, no other means of transportation and who, because of the severity of their disabilities, or distance, would be unable to use public transportation.

The center attempted to meet transportation needs through its own resources, in addition to leasing a bus. However, the effort was merely a stopgap, and the need was there to develop an efficient, safe, and well-coordinated transportation system if services to the clientele were not to be reduced or impaired. Such a system was developed and included several nine-passenger station wagons, a hydraulic lift equipped bus, and a more effective, well-coordinated route.

The facility, having committed all of its resources, found that the transportation system which was so necessary was unobtainable unless additional help was secured. Consequently, a facilities improvement grant request was submitted to the Division of Vocational Rehabilitation for the needed equipment. It was approved; the equipment was purchased, and the vital link between the home where the client lives and the hope of rehabilitation was sustained.

By using the federal grants where needed and seeing that they were distributed fairly across the state, a modern and effective system for rehabilitation services has become a reality. The federal grants which in 1968 amounted to $1,005,952 have been used effectively, so that today with a slightly reduced expenditure of federal money amounting to $401,000, this network of private centers can still increase its services to clients, and in particular, severely disabled people.[7]

The Rehabilitation Facilities and Division of Vocational Rehabilitation in Connecticut have had remarkable support from business and industry with the help of the Governor's Committee on Employment of the Handicapped, state and local Chambers of Commerce, The Manufacturers Association, Human Relations Commission, labor unions, the Department of Labor and other public and private community agencies. They have been extremely successful in obtaining subcontractual work from business and industry. Some examples of companies who have had management personnel who arranged to get subcontract work to the workshops are: (1) Waring Products (2) Pitney Bowes, Inc. (3) Torrington Company (4) Scoville Manufacturing Company (5) Fafnir Bearing Company (6) Electric Boat Division of General Dynamics (7) United Technologies (8) Carling Electric (9) Valve Corporation of America (10) Remington Arms (11) Producto Machines (12) Southern New England Telephone Company (13) Sargent Tool Company.

In Connecticut we continue to foster the premise that there are at least two overall objectives to which all workshops can subscribe. These objectives are made clear, as far as possible, to the client, the workshop and the community.

"One objective of the workshop is the rehabilitation of the handicapped individual; the other is the services to the community in meeting the needs of its handicapped population."[3]

Effectiveness of the Partnership

To show the effectiveness of public/private cooperation, one need only look to the great increase that has taken place in the last eight years. In 1968 there were only 41 rehabilitation facilities statewide. Now there are over 51 such facilities, many having satellites at various locations in their region. These new facilities and their satellites are also strategically located to make services closer to all potential clients.

The number of DVR funded clients served by rehabilitation facilities has increased dramatically from approximately 1,732 in 1968 to approximately 2,353 during 1975—a 35.8% increase.[4] This increase for DVR clients is also mirrored in the Title 110 monies spent. In 1958, $613,024 was expended while during 1975 over $827,019 was spent, a percentage increase of 34.7. The above comparisons demonstrate the very efficient way in which the rehabilitation center system in Connecticut has been expanded and utilized (see map).

Through mutual planning and effective use of grants and other resources over the years, Connecticut now has a rehabilitation facilities system with the ability to provide quality services to clientele throughout the state. This is not a static system, however, for the partnership realizes the need to provide more comprehensive services to more severely disabled individuals on a larger scale. Consequently, there are ongoing reviews and needs assessment to help insure that future developments within the system will continue to have synergistic effect, so that all will benefit, especially the clients.

The general objective of our Comprehensive Statewide Planning for Vocational Rehabilitation Workshops and Facilities, which was published in 1970, was to develop a plan for workshops and rehabilitation facilities for meeting the needs of Connecticut's disabled citizens by 1975. The above plan proved simple, flexible, and practical. By and large, the ten (10) recommendations resulting from this study have been met. This represents a major accomplishment by the DVR agency in conjunction with the support and cooperation of many other agencies and people. Recommendations (1) (2) and (6) are worthy of review.

Recommendation 1

There is a critical need for the broader type of services provided by rehabilitation centers with workshops. These services can be furnished by the expansion of smaller facilities in the Waterbury and Norwich regions or the construction of new facilities.

The presently established centers in Bridgeport, New Haven, and Hartford should examine the possibilities of operating satellite centers in adjacent geographic areas.

Recommendation 2

Seven additional rehabilitation facilities with primary emphasis on the full range of vocational training services, including extended employment, oriented to disabilities other than mental retardation should be located in the following:

1. Hartford Region   (1)
2. New Haven Region   (2)
3. Waterbury Region   (2)
4. Norwich Region   (2)

Recommendation 6

The small faculties in the state should be encouraged and guided in their efforts to expand their physical facilities and the professional capabilities of their staffs.[5]

"At this point in time," to use a current politically flavored phraseology, we do not presume that our partnership effort is done. Although we have brought rehabilitation facilities within useful range of nearly every handicapped (1975 estimate, 180,000+) citizen, we still fall short of our goal of making rehabilitation services available to all of the state's disabled citizens who can profit from services. We must, however, double our efforts so that by the year 2000, this goal will be a reality. It is our prediction that such a grandiose accomplishment will take about 25 years, but "we can make it if we try!"

In our study of the vocational rehabilitation delivery system of 14 Western European Countries and Yugoslavia, we found varying degrees of similarities and differences. There is little or not uniformity, with the possible exception of a deep concern for disabled and disadvantaged people. Officials and functionaries of both private and public agencies agree that vocational rehabilitation, like health, social security, workmen's compensation, education, etc., is a right of the people that the country concerned had to recognize. In every country visited, this idea was the prevailing principle enacted by law and statute. Undergirding the law and statue is a humanitarian philosophy of service to people in order to foster independent living and avoid dependency.[6] It is through such a frame of reference that we have developed our successful partnership in rehabilitation in the Constitution State—Connecticut.

References

1. Chouinard, Edward L. and Garrett, James F., Editors. *Workshop for the Disabled. A Vocational Rehabilitation Resource.* U.S. Department of Health, Education, and Welfare. Office of Vocational Rehabilitation, Washington, D.C., 1956.

2. Connecticut State Division of Vocational Rehabilitation: *Annual Report.* Hartford, Connecticut, 1968-69.

3. Connecticut State Division of Vocational Rehabilitation: *Annual Report.* Hartford, Connecticut, 1969-70.

4. Connecticut State Board of Education: *Evaluations and Reports as Mandated by the General Assembly.* Hartford, Connecticut, Feb. 1975.

5. Peters, II, James S. and Prior, Albert C., *Final Report Comprehensive Statewide Planning for Vocational Rehabilitation Workshops and Facilities.* Volume IV, Hartford, Connecticut, 1970.

6. Peters, II, James S. *Vocational Rehabilitation of the Disabled and Disadvantaged in the United States and Europe.* The American School for the Deaf, West Hartford, Connecticut, 1975.

7. Public Law 90-391, 30th Congress 1 & R 16819 amendments of 1968, Section 12.

8. Thompson, Nellie Z., Editor, *the Role of the Workshop in Rehabilitation, Office of Vocational Rehabilitation,* U.S. Department of Health, Education and Welfare, Washington, D.C., July 1955.

❦

CHAPTER TWENTY-ONE

RIGHTS OF THE HANDICAPPED

James S. Peters, II, Ph.D.
Storrs, Connecticut

I am pleased to be a part of this panel, "Endowed by Their Creator: Human Rights in the World Today," sponsored by Bahaïs of Norwich, an organization whose ideas and philosophy I have admired through the years. Let me indulge your patience by quoting from a standard Bahaï writing:

> In the sight of God there is no distinction between whites and blacks; all are as one. Anyone whose heart is pure is dear to God-whether white or black, red or yellow. Among the animals color exist. The doves are white, black, red, blue; but not withstanding this diversity of color they flock together...Man is intelligent and thoughtful, endowed with powers of mind. Why then should he be influenced by distinction of color or race, since all belong to one human family?

So be it with the physically and mentally handicapped or disabled among us, they have their rights as members of the human family.

"Social justice for the Disabled" reflects the basic orientation of the field of Vocational Rehabilitation with its focus on the dignity of persons, enhanced self-esteem, and independence. These are all fine words, but the Rehabilitation Movement in Connecticut and in the United States has matched these words by actions, along with positive changes and the development of a network of vital resources to serve the multiplicity of needs in the rehabilitation process.

A talk given at Human Rights Day Panel discussion by the Bahais of Norwich, Connecticut, Thames Valley Technical College, Saturday, December 10, 1988.

Many new challenges were met as new laws expanded the mandate of Rehabilitation programs in the country. These new initiatives stressed mentally impaired, emotionally disturbed persons, as well as those with alcohol and drug disabilities, and the public offender. The Consumer Rights Movement added a new and vital dimension to the work of the State Vocational Rehabilitation System in serving persons with the most severe problems.

The state-federal rehabilitation agency in Connecticut is the Division of Vocational Rehabilitation of the State Department of Education. Throughout its years of service (1930-1980) to the handicapped it has maintained unusual stability concurrent with remarkable change. Aside from a few periods when other senior staff members took charge temporarily, wile the Directors' efforts were divided to broaden issues, there have been only two administrators for the program. From the time the State enabling legislation was passed in 1929 Edward P. Chester, the first agency head, whose tenure began in September 1930, guided the fortunes of rehabilitation until August 1956. Beginning in August 1956 until July 1981 James S. Peters, II was administrator. With remarkable adaptability, the program has ranged outward from a modest effort serving the orthopedically disabled with emphasis on workmen's compensation cases. Over the years, it added services to assist individuals handicapped by disabling conditions running the gamut from orthopedic to congenital to mental and even, for a time, behavioral disorders. To add perspective to this management stability during the same span of time, there have been six Commissioners of Education and fourteen Governors of the State of Connecticut.

The history of the Division of Vocational Rehabilitation in Connecticut largely follows the prevailing trends of its social milieu. Differences in goals and approaches to the problems of handicapping conditions affected both the professional rehabilitation counselors and their clients. Even these were altered by the resources—often scanty—at hand to accomplish the basic purpose. In 1919, Gerard Harris, author of *The Redemption of the Disabled*, (1919)—probably the earliest book on rehabilitation—held the fundamental aim to be "a demand for social justice which no democracy can deny," and the "avoidance of dependency." In variant forms this was the germ of the ideal for rehabilitation here as elsewhere, social justice for the handicapped.

Throughout its history, the agency has been client centered, frequently in spite of a social environment not conducive to this approach. The handicapped individuals served by the agency have evolved from a relatively passive population to one taking a healthy activist role, asserting their rights under the federal Rehabilitation Act of 1973. The result can only be a healthier relationship between the rehabilitation agency and the people it serves. The narration of this Golden Anniversary of Vocational Rehabilitation flushed out the evolution of this constructive effort. The continuing drama of the conflict between cost and "the demand for social justice" for the handicapped is evident in these times.

Fiscal 1970 (July 1, 1969 to June 30, 1970 embraced the 50th anniversary of vocational rehabilitation nationally. Connecticut';s program had advanced from the one-person operation of the 1930s and the three-person program of 1940 to a total of 97 professional working with 10,635 handicapped individuals. Basic ideas of what was being done had advanced from the early emphasis upon guidance, training and placement to the view of the individual as a whole, and the provision of services for that whole being. Individual needs for a wide variety of services had been demonstrated over the years. The 1970s were to be the decade of consumer rights and consumer activism. Society's frequently reiterated and proven economic reasons for restoring the handicapped to independence were being accepted. Theoretically, an advanced civilization such as ours could order itself so that all disabled individuals so far as possible might have the right to dignity and independence. The consumers of rehabilitation services, the handicapped citizens of the State of Connecticut, would be pressing politically, for these rights envisioned as just those qualities of dignity and independence.

In our investigation of the Vocational Rehabilitation delivery system of fourteen Western European Countries and Yugoslavia we found varying degrees of similarities and differences. There is little or no uniformity, with the possible exception of a deep concern for the disabled and disadvantaged. In discussing this concern with many government officials and functionaries of public and private agencies we were informed that vocational rehabilitation was a right of the people that the country concerned had to recognize. Vocational rehabilitation, like health, social security, workmen's compensation, education, etc., is, potentially, welfare, available for all who are in need and who can profit therefrom. In every country visited this was the prevailing principle enacted by law and statute. Undergirding the law and statute, so it seems, is a humanitarian philosophy of service to people in order to foster independent living and avoid dependency.

It was quite evident that vocational rehabilitation is a Federal government responsibility. Private efforts are encouraged, and in many instances the private health and charity organizations play a leadership role in the development of new programs and provide for their funding. But in the final analysis, it is the Federal government that furnishes the muscles which, frequently in partnership with the private sector, enables handicapped and disadvantaged citizens to receive vocational rehabilitation through the various services and facilities available.

In the United States we have the Federal government in partnership with the states fostering vocational rehabilitation services in a more structured manner, it appears, than in the European countries we visited. Other public and private health, welfare, labor, educational, and industrial organizations work very closely with the state operations and the results are similar to those found in Europe. It seems that among our professional and volunteer workers the aims and objectives are the same, i.e., helping the handicapped become more independent in our society. But, still, a basic problem here in the United States is making rehabilitation services available to all of those in need and who could, therefore, benefit from these services.

It is a recognizable fact that compared with the European countries visited, the United States is monstrous in size and population, as well as diverse in its people and customs. We must also be reminded of the fact that institutional, religious, and racial prejudice has frustrated past efforts to extend vocational rehabilitation services, as well as other humanitarian services; to the poor, blacks, and other minorities. Then, too, our country and its civilian population was not harmed directly by two World Wars. This, in and of itself, has had, it seems to us an enlightening effect upon the people of Europe and their national government. Perhaps there is a greater appreciation of the needs of the handicapped for it is closer to home. Rehabilitation workshops and facilities are pointed to with pride, and the government gives financial support, etc. to many of them. Industry is expected to, and does, work closely with the government in training and providing employment on a full- or part-time basis for the handicapped. In Europe this relationship is mandated, in the United States it is permissive.

Because of the limited time spent in each country and the, by necessity, superficial observation of workshops and rehabilitation centers and their impact on vocational rehabilitation effort in the United States and in Europe, our recommendations are few but pervasive. They are the following:

1. Develop a vocational rehabilitation program where the Federal government will be responsible for its delivery system. The states could be reimbursed 90 to 100% of cost. Through this type of organization, all handicapped individuals, potentially, could be served.
2. Increase the client service capacity of the state vocational

rehabilitation agencies by allowing all counseling, consulting, coordinating, etc. efforts, to receive credit, as well as the number of rehabilitants (number placed in productive employment.)

3. Make funds available in the form of grants to all certified rehabilitation centers and workshops that are providing services to the handicapped in the United States.

4. Appropriate funds for building of rehabilitation workshops and facilities on a non matching basis, similar to methods used by Department of Hosing and Redevelopment but without the repayment feature.

❦

THE AUTHOR

James S. Peters, II received his Ph.D. in counseling and clinical psychology from Purdue University where he was a Veterans Administration Fellow and Research Associate. His undergraduate degree was completed at Southern University, Baton Rouge, Louisiana. At Southern he was a T.H. Harris Scholarship Fellow, Captain, and Little All-American football player. He holds a Master of Arts Degree in Social Psychology from the Hartford Seminary Foundation; Master of Science Degree, Clinical Psychology, Illinois Institute of Technology; and has done graduate work in Psychology at the University of Chicago, where he was a clinical psychology intern in the Veterans Administration program. At the present time he is an independent practitioner of psychology. For 25 years he was Associate Commissioner, Division of Vocational Rehabilitation and Disability Determination, Connecticut State Department of Education; Adjunct Professor, Department of Psychology, University of Hartford; and Lecturer on rehabilitation, Department of Educational Psychology, University of Connecticut. Dr. Peters is a licensed psychologist in the states of Connecticut, New York, New Hampshire, Massachusetts, Vermont, California, and certified in Louisiana. During 1971-1973 he was a Postdoctoral Research Fellow, Harvard University, School of Medicine, Department of Psychiatry, and a Special Fellow of the U.S., Department of Health, Education, and Welfare, Social and Rehabilitation Services, while studying rehabilitation in the United States and Europe. In 1976 and 1977 he studied rehabilitation needs in West Africa and Brazil.

Prior to Dr. Peters' appointment to administer Vocational Rehabilitation in Connecticut he was Director of Graduate Training in Rehabilitation Counseling and Assistant Professor of Psychology at Springfield College (Massachusetts). In addition, he had been a high school teacher and counselor in Louisiana, clinical and counseling psychologist with the Veterans Administration in the Chicago area, and a specialist-teacher (psychologist) with the U. S. Navy during World War II.

During the spring semester of 1984-1985 at Southern University, his alma mater, he was Visiting Professor of Psychology, and Rehabilitation Counseling, Department of Psychology. In 1977-1978 he was "Distinguished Visiting Professor of Rehabilitation," Southern Illinois University at Carbondale. There he assisted in establishing the doctoral rehabilitation program—the country's first.

In 1999 Dr. Peters was awarded Diplomate Status by the American Psychotherapy Association in recognition of his personal integrity and professional accomplishments.

www.ingramcontent.com/pod-product-compliance
Lightning Source LLC
Chambersburg PA
CBHW062036270326
41929CB00014B/2445